T0212117

Lecture Notes in Computer Science 11850

More information about this series at http://www.springer.com/series/7412

Dan Nguyen · Lei Xing · Steve Jiang (Eds.)

Artificial Intelligence in Radiation Therapy

First International Workshop, AIRT 2019
Held in Conjunction with MICCAI 2019
Shenzhen, China, October 17, 2019
Proceedings

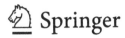 Springer

Editors
Dan Nguyen ⓘ
The University of Texas
Southwestern Medical Center
Dallas, TX, USA

Lei Xing
Stanford University
Stanford, CA, USA

Steve Jiang
The University of Texas
Southwestern Medical Center
Dallas, TX, USA

ISSN 0302-9743   ISSN 1611-3349 (electronic)
Lecture Notes in Computer Science
ISBN 978-3-030-32485-8   ISBN 978-3-030-32486-5   (eBook)
https://doi.org/10.1007/978-3-030-32486-5

LNCS Sublibrary: SL6 – Image Processing, Computer Vision, Pattern Recognition, and Graphics

This Springer imprint is published by the registered company Springer Nature Switzerland AG
The registered company address is: Gewerbestrasse 11, 6330 Cham, Switzerland

Preface

We are pleased to present the proceedings to the First International Workshop for Artificial Intelligence in Radiation Therapy (AIRT 2019), which took place on October 17, 2019, and was held in conjunction with the 22nd International Conference on Medical Image Computing and Computer Assisted Intervention (MICCAI 2019), in Shenzhen, China, during October 13–17, 2019.

This workshop included 20 accepted presentations featuring the most recent work focused on the application of artificial intelligence (AI) and automation technologies in radiation therapy. With this workshop, we hope to open a discussion about the state of radiation therapy, the state of AI and related technologies, and pave the way to revolutionizing the field to ultimately improve cancer patient outcome and quality of life. We believe that in working with the intelligent minds at MICCAI, the field of radiation therapy will greatly benefit from the exposure of the latest cutting-edge algorithms, and MICCAI will grow from tackling the unique challenges in radiation therapy.

In particular, we will focus on the application and development of AI and related technologies in two fronts: (1) image guided treatment delivery and (2) image guided treatment strategy. Image guided treatment delivery will be focused on advancements of technologies that are used during the delivery of the radiation to the patient for image guided radiation therapy (IGRT), which includes developments in cone beam computed tomography (CBCT), fluoroscopy, surface imaging, motion management, and other modalities that are used for IGRT. Image guided treatment strategy will involve technologies that are used in the clinical pipeline leading up to the delivery, which include segmentation techniques and algorithms on CT, MRI, and/or PET, treatment planning, dose calculation, quality assurance and error detection, etc.

CBCT, fluoroscopy, surface imaging, and related submissions for image guided treatment delivery focus on the use of the imaging modalities for accurate and precise delivery of the planned radiation dose onto the tumor and healthy tissue. Motion management includes immobilization methods and imaging for motion verification or prediction. Segmentation related submissions focus on the segmentation that is specific to the radiotherapy pipeline, and may use CT, MRI, and/or PET images for algorithm development. Treatment planning submissions focus on techniques and algorithms for improving the plan quality and/or the planning efficiency. Dose calculation related submissions focus on photon, electron, protons, or heavy ion, with applications to radiation therapy. Quality assurance and error detection submissions relate to ensuring that the calculated dose matches the delivered dose, identifying human mistakes during treatment planning and delivery, incident learning, risk analysis, and process control.

We employed the EasyChair[1] conference management system for our paper submissions and peer review process. Any identifying information was redacted in the

---

[1] https://easychair.org/

submission prior to review to maintain an anonymous review process. In total, 24 full submissions were received and the overall acceptance rate was 83.3%. The accepted papers have been compiled into a volume of *Lecture Notes in Computer Science* (LNCS) proceedings—Volume LNCS 11850.

We would like to thank everyone who contributed greatly to the success of AIRT 2019 and the quality of its proceedings, especially the authors, co-authors, students, and supervisors, for submitting and presenting their exceptional work to the AIRT workshop. We believe that this workshop for AI in radiation therapy is the perfect platform for providing discussion of the state of radiation therapy, the state of AI and related technologies, and will pave the way to revolutionizing the field to ultimately improve cancer patient outcome and quality of life.

September 2019

Dan Nguyen
Lei Xing
Steve Jiang

Organization

Organizing Committee

Dan Nguyen — Medical Artificial Intelligence and Automation (MAIA) Laboratory, Department of Radiation Oncology, UT Southwestern Medical Center, USA

Lei Xing — Laboratory for Artificial Intelligence in Medicine and Biomedical Physics, Department of Radiation Oncology, Stanford Medicine, USA

Steve Jiang — Medical Artificial Intelligence and Automation (MAIA) Laboratory, Department of Radiation Oncology, UT Southwestern Medical Center, USA

Contents

Using Supervised Learning and Guided Monte Carlo Tree Search for Beam Orientation Optimization in Radiation Therapy

Azar Sadeghnejad Barkousaraie, Olalekan Ogunmolu, Steve Jiang, and Dan Nguyen$^{(\boxtimes)}$

Medical Artificial Intelligence and Automation (MAIA) Laboratory, Department of Radiation Oncology, University of Texas Southwestern Medical Center, Dallas, TX 75390, USA
{Azar.Barkousaraie, Olalekan.Ogunmolu, Steve.Jiang, Dan.Nguyen}@utsouthwestern.edu

Abstract. In clinical practice, the beam orientation selection process is either tediously done by the planner or based on specific protocols, typically yielding suboptimal and inefficient solutions. Column generation (CG) has been shown to produce superior plans compared to those of human selected beams, especially in highly non-coplanar plans such as 4π Radiotherapy. In this work, we applied AI to explore the decision space of beam orientation selection. At first, a supervised deep learning neural network (SL) is trained to mimic a CG generated policy. By iteratively using SL to predict the next beam, a set of beam orientations would be selected. However, iteratively using SL to select the next beam does not guarantee the plan's quality. Although the teacher policy, CG, is an efficient method, it is a greedy algorithm and still finds suboptimal solutions that are subject to improvement. To address this, a reinforcement learning application of guided Monte Carlo tree search (GTS) was implemented, coupled with SL to guide the traversal through the tree, and update the fitness values of its nodes. To test the feasibility of GTS, 13 test prostate cancer patients were evaluated. Our results show that we maintained a similar planning target volume (PTV) coverage within 2% error margin, reduce the organ at risk (OAR) mean dose, and in general improve the objective function value, while decreasing the computation time.

Keywords: Radiation therapy · Prostate cancer · IMRT · Beam orientation · Monte Carlo Tree Search · Artificial intelligent · Deep neural network

1 Introduction

In intensity-modulated radiation therapy (IMRT), the optimal choice of beam orientations has a significant impact on the treatment plan quality, influencing the final treatment outcome. In current treatment planning workflow, the beam orientations are either manually selected by the planner in a tedious fashion, or chosen based on specific protocols, typically yielding suboptimal solutions. Beam Orientation Optimization (BOO) methods are used to find the optimal beam directions. Due to the

© Springer Nature Switzerland AG 2019
D. Nguyen et al. (Eds.): AIRT 2019, LNCS 11850, pp. 1–9, 2019.
https://doi.org/10.1007/978-3-030-32486-5_1

highly combinatorial nature of the BOO problem, many optimization algorithms have employed heuristics to approximate its solution. One of the successful algorithms specially for solving complex and highly non-coplanar problems such as 4π radiotherapy [1] is Column Generation (CG). While efficient, CG is a greedy algorithm and typically finds suboptimal solutions. In this work we first present the CG implementation for BOO problem, where CG iteratively solves a sequence of Fluence Map Optimization (FMO) [2] problems by using GPU-based Chambolle-Pock algorithm. Then a Monte Carlo Tree Search subsequently improves the quality of BOO solution. However, CG is a time intensive operation, therefore we propose a deep neural network that learns the decision process of the CG policy and is able to solve BOO problem in less than one second for a 5-beam IMRT plan. Then we used this supervised deep learning approach to guide the decision tree faster. The proposed beam orientation optimization framework is capable of finding a superior solution over CG, in less amount of time.

2 Methods

The proposed method has a reinforcement learning structure involving a supervised learning network to guide Monte Carlo tree search to explore the beam orientation selection decision space. This method, guided Monte Carlo tree search, consists of two components: Monte Carlo Tree Search (MCTS) as the main structure of the method and supervised learning network (SL) as a guidance policy network, to traverse the decision tree search faster. In this section, brief description of key terms and algorithms in the proposed method are provided.

- *Patient Anatomical Features:* include the images of cancer patients with contoured structures and treatment planning weights assigned to each structure. The images of 70 prostate cancer patients are used for this research, each with 6 contours, PTV, body, bladder, rectum, and left and right femoral heads. The weights assigned to the structures are chosen randomly.
- *State of the problem:* include patient's anatomical features and a set of selected beam orientations (B). At the beginning of the planning, this set has no member, and it is updated throughout the solution procedure.
- *Actions:* The selection of the next beam orientation to be added to set B, given the state of the problem.
- *Solution or terminal state*: state of the problem in which the number of selected beam orientations (size of B) is the same as a predefined number of beams, chosen by user. At this point, a feasible solution for the problem is generated.
- *Cost or objective function*: $\min_x \frac{1}{2}\sum_{s \in S} w_s^2 \|D_s x - p\|_2^2$ s.t. $x \geq 0$, where w_s is the structure weight for structure s, $D_s x$ the amount of dose received by structure s, and p is the prescription dose.
- *Beam fitness values*: produced by the calculations of optimality conditions based on the objective function. Fitness value of a beam (b_i) shows the possible improvement in the objective function by adding b_i to set B.

2.1   Column Generation

The SL network learns from an optimization process (Column Generation) to find the suitable beam orientation for each state of the problem. In the proposed Column Generation (CG), after FMO of a given state of the problem is solved by the Chambolle-Pock algorithm [3], CG calculates the fitness values of all candidate beams. These values are generated by using Karush-Kuhn-Tucker (KKT) conditions for optimality [4, 5]. Given a state of the problem, CG finds the next best beam to be added to the current set of selected beam orientations B, such that adding this beam will improve the cost function the most. The whole process of iteratively solving FMO, calculating fitness values, selecting the next beam and updating the state of the problem, is called CG in this paper.

Although CG is a powerful optimization tool, itis computationally expensive and requires many resources (time, computational resources and calculation of dose influence matrices of all candidate beams). Using SL network instead of Column Generation (CG) helps to find a set of good beam orientations quickly, with limited resources and available information. The structure of the supervised training process is shown in Fig. 1. The beamlet dose data in this figure represents dose influence matrices of each possible beamlet among all candidate beams for every structure of each patient, which its calculation needs few hours at least. After SL is trained by CG solutions, beamlet dose data is not required for solving beam orientation optimization. Note that at the end to find the best arrangement of the selected beams, dose influence matrices of the selected beams should be calculated and FMO problem should be solved. But in this case, dose influence matrices of only those selected beam orientations is required, for example in this project, the dose influence calculation of five beams is required compared to the total 180 candidate beams available.

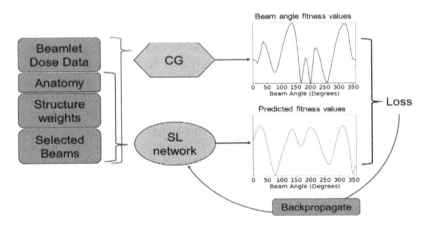

Fig. 1. Schematic of the Supervised Training Structure to predict Beam Orientation fitness values. Column Generation (CG) as teacher and deep neural (SL) as Trainee.

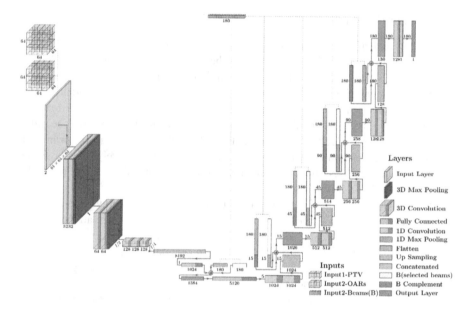

Fig. 2. Proposed deep learning neural network structure. (Color figure online)

2.2   Supervised Deep Learning Neural Network

The network architecture of the proposed SL is shown in Fig. 2, and designed as a sequence of 3-D and 1-D convolutional (orange-colored in Fig. 2), max-pooling (Red), flatten (yellow), fully connected (purple), concatenation (green) and up-sampling (light blue) layers. The SL inputs are the anatomical structures, namely PTV and Organs at Risk or OARs (pink and blue cubes), and set B (purple). The output (blue-green array) is an array of size 180 (number of potential beam orientations) that represents the fitness values or the probability of success in choosing a beam orientation.

The SL network has three blocks of layers. In the first block, the patient's anatomy is analyzed, while the set of already selected beams, or *Input2* array, is fed into the second and third blocks of layers as two arrays B and its complement[1] B^C. In second block, arrays B and B^C, are merged to the 1-dimensional convolution layer from first block. In each stage of the third block of layers, max-polling layer of second input arrays, are added to the up-sampled 1D convolutional layers. After the last convolution layer, there is only one feature array of size 180. This array represents the fitness value of each beam orientation, as the possible changes to the current objective function (current solution) or probability of success.

The activation functions of all the layers in the proposed model are Scaled Exponential Linear Unit (SELU). SELU is a self-normalizing activation function, which is proven to converge to zero mean and unit variance even under the presence of

---

[1] x and y are complemented, if $x \vee y = 1, x \wedge y = 0$

noises, and makes learning robust even for deep neural networks with so many layers [6]. The loss function of the model is Mean Squared Error (MSE) with Adam optimizer with learning rate of 10^{-5}.

Algorithm 1.a: *Iterative structure of CG to select N beams for one patient*

```
1. Initialize B as an empty array
2. Set current number of selected beam orientations in B as 0,
   N_B = 0
3. Calculate D_ij for all beamlets (j) of all potential beams (i)
4. While N_B < N, do:
   a. Solve FMO associated to B with Chambolle-Pock Algorithm
   b. Calculate potential fitness values
   c. Set b* as beam orientation with maximum fitness value b* ∉ B
   d. B = B ∪ {b*}, N_B = N_B +1
5.  Return B
```

Algorithm 1.b: *Iterative structure of SL to select N beams for one patient*

```
1. Initialize B as an empty array
2. Set current number of beam orientations in B as 0, N_B = 0
3. While N_B < N , do:
   a. Use SL to predict the next beam (b*)
   b. B = B ∪ {b*}, N_B = N_B +1
4. Return B
```

The trained SL is used to predict the solution of BOO. The iterative structure of CG and SL are shown in and Algorithm 1a and b respectively, where differences are highlited by red) The images of 70 prostate cancer patients, each with 6 contours, are used to train and test the network. 57 patients are considered for training and validation in a 6-fold cross validation technique and 13 paitent for test set. All six models are trained over 400 epochs each with 2500 steps. From each fold, the trained model with least validation loss function (Mean Squared Error) was selected and used for prediction on the test set.

2.3   Monte Carlo Tree Search

Monte Carlo Tree Search (MCTS) uses the decision tree to explore the decision space, by randomly sampling from it [7]. The search process of MCTS consists of four steps, node selection, expansion, simulation and backpropagation on the simulation result. In this work, each node represents a beam orientation and each branch from root to its leaves are the selected sets of beams. It means the depth of the tree is the same as the number of beam orientations in the solution set. The details of each process and general algorithm are presented in Algorithm 2.

The pretrained SL, probabilistically guides the traversal of the branches on the Monte Carlo decision tree to add a new beam to the plan. A search of a plan starts from root, as an empty set of beam, and contintues until it reaches the terminal state. After the exploration of each complete plan, the fluence map optimization problem is solved and based on that, the probability distribution to select next beam will be updated, using the reward function, in backpropagation stage. Then starting from root again, the exploring of the next branch will start, untill the stopping criteria is met.

Algorithm 2. *Select N beam orientations from M candidate beams*

1. Initialize B as an empty array, $BestCostValue = \infty$ and $BestBeamSelection = \emptyset$
2. Create a root node R, $R_{name} = 'Root'$
3. Set D_R as an array of fitness values for each beam, predicted by NN given no selected beams $|B| = 0$
4. Set current node $(NC = R)$ and stop = False
5. While stop == False
   a. Choose the next beam (b_{next}) as a randomly generated variable with probability distribution of D_{NC}.
   b. Add b_{next} to B and Set nodename = NC_{name} + '-' + b_{next}
   c. If NC does not have a child named as **nodename** :
      (1) Create node Nnew with $Nnew_{name} = nodename$, $Nnew_{parent} = NC$ and add Nnew to $NC_{children}$ and set $Nnew_{visit} = 1$
      (2) Set D_{Nnew} as a predicted fitness values using SL given set B, and Set $NC = Nnew_{name}$.
   d. Else:
      (1) Set NC as NC_{child} with name **nodename**, $Nnew_{visit} += 1$
   e. If $|B| == N$:
      (1) Solve FMO given set B and save the cost value $Cost_{now}$ as NC_{cost}
      (2) If $BestCostValue > NC_{cost}$:
         i. Set $BestCostValue = NC_{cost}$, $BestBeamSelection = B$, $NC_{reward} = 1$.
      (3) Else:
         i. $NC_{reward} = \frac{(BestCostValue - NC_{cost})}{NC_{cost}} + 0.15$
      (4) While $NC \neq R$:
         i. $NC = NC_{parent}$, $NC_{reward} = \frac{\sum_{CH \in NC_{children}} CH_{rewards}}{|NC_{chilren}|}$,
         ii. $D_{NC}[b_{next}] = \frac{D_{NC}[b_{next}]}{NC_{visit}} + NC_{reward}$
         iii. If $NC_{cost} > Cost_{now}$: $NC_{cost} = Cost_{now}$
      (5) $B = \infty$, $D_{NC} = D_R$
   f. If stopping criteria is met: Stop = True
6. Return $BestCostValue, BestBeamSelection$

---

3 Results and Discussion

More than 3000 input scenarios for training, validating and testing the SL network were generated, by randomly assigning structure weights and image rotations. The average and standard deviation of train, validation and test loss functions among all folds were $0.62 \pm 0.09\%$, $1.04 \pm 0.06\%$, and $1.44 \pm 0.11\%$ respectively. Trained model with least validation loss function was used for final comparision. By using CG and SL, two sets of beam orientations for each scenario in test set were selected, and their associated FMOs were solved. In terms up just solving the BOO problem, SL took under 1.5 s for a 5 beam prediction while column generation took more than 10 min to solve for its beam orentations. Since SL only needs dose calculation on its 5 chosen beams, the whole process takes an average of 5 min 20 s, as opposed to the 3 h CG needs to calculated the doses of all 180 candidate beams. The values of six metrics, which have been used to compare treatment plans created by CG and SL, is presented in Table 1 (metrics definition in [8]). Bladder had the minimum average differences in dose recieved by OARs (0.956 ± 1.184) and Right Femoral head had the maximum (5.885 ± 5.515). The differences in the dose coverage of PTV between CG and SL plans were 0.2%, while the average dose differences recieved by organs at risk were between 1 to 6%, $0.10 \pm 0.1\%$ (body), $1.06 \pm 1.42\%$ (bladder), $2.44 \pm 2.11\%$ (rectum), $6.03 \pm 5.86\%$ (L fem head), $6.38 \pm 5.94\%$ (R fem head).

Table 1. Mean $\pm$ standard deviation for PTV Statistics, van't Riet Conformation Number (VR), and High Dose Spillage (R50) Metrics values of CG and SL beam set of test dataset.

	CG results	SL prediction	Diff CG-SL
PTV D98	0.977 ± 0.011	0.976 ± 0.012	0.00 ± 0.003
PTV D99	0.961 ± 0.020	0.960 ± 0.020	0.001 ± 0.005
PTV Dmax	0.87 ± 0.059	0.87 ± 0.057	0.00 ± 0.031
PTV Homogeneity	0.069 ± 0.038	0.070 ± 0.038	-0.001 ± 0.004
VR	0.881 ± 0.083	0.879 ± 0.093	0.002 ± 0.021
R50	4.676 ± 0.888	4.555 ± 0.694	0.121 ± 0.372

Then the selected trained SL model was used as the guidance policy in GTS. On average, the CG algorithm needed 700 s to solve FMO of an iteratively augmented problem to select 5 beams, while the proposed GTS found solutions with higher

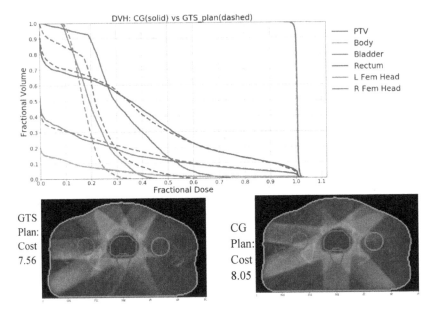

Fig. 3. CG generated plan (solid) vs GTS generated plan (dashed)

quality, with respect to the objective value, in 100 s on average. Scenarios of test dataset (13 patients) were used to test the quality of GTS solution compare to CG. Using GTS method, we were able to maintain a similar planning targe volume (PTV) coverage within 2% error (D98 = 0.97 ± 0.01 and D99 = 0.95 ± 0.02), and **reduce** the organ at risk (OAR) mean dose by 0.10 ± 0.08% (body), 2.44 ± 2.01% (rectum), 4.94 ± 4.65% (L fem head), 6.40 ± 3.94% (R fem head), of the prescription dose, but a slight increase of 1.31 ± 1.96% in bladder. A test patient's plans generated by CG and GTS is presented in Fig. 3. Although the presented method is good enough but it still has room for improvement (e.g. bladder dose), and future more detailed study to improve the algorithm is planned.

4 Conclusion

In this study, first we proposed a supervised deep neural network (SL) to learn column generation (CG) decision-making process, and predict the fitness values of all candidate beams, beam with maximum fitness value will be chosen to add to the solution. CG although powerful, is a heuristic, greedy algorithm that cannot guarantee the optimality of the final solution, and it leaves room for improvement, so a Monte Carlo guided tree search (GTS) is proposed to see if finding a solution with better objective function in reasonable amount of time is feasible. After SL is trained, it is used to generate the beams fitness values for nodes in the decision tree, where each node represents a set of selected beams. Fitness values in each node are normalized and used as probability mass function (PMF) to help deciding decision tree extension. Later PFM will be modified by reward function, which is based on the final objective values of solving FMO for every five selected beams. GTS continues to explore the decision tree until at least one of the resources (time, average improvement, etc.) is exhausted. We demonstrate that suggested GTS method produces a superior plan to CG in reducing the objective value, in less time than it takes to solve the CG algorithm. Considering the success of GTS in reducing the objective function and its potential for further improvement, we will continue exploring new methods and techniques to upgrade the quality of treatment planning with the help of artificial intelligence.

References

1. Dong, P., et al.: 4π noncoplanar stereotactic body radiation therapy for centrally located or larger lung tumors. Int. J. Radiat. Oncol.* Biol.* Phys. **86**, 407–413 (2013)
2. Cabrera-Guerrero, G., Lagos, C., Cabrera, E., Johnson, F., Rubio, J.M., Paredes, F.: Comparing local search algorithms for the beam angles selection in radiotherapy. IEEE Access **6**, 23701–23710 (2018)
3. Chambolle, A., Pock, T.: A first-order primal-dual algorithm for convex problems with applications to imaging. J. Math. Imaging Vis. **40**, 120–145 (2011)
4. Kuhn, H., Tucker, A.: Proceedings of 2nd Berkeley Symposium. University of California Press, Berkeley (1951)

5. Karush, W.: Minima of functions of several variables with inequalities as side conditions. In: Giorgi, G., Kjeldsen, T.H. (eds.) Traces and Emergence of Nonlinear Programming, pp. 217–245. Springer, Basel (2014). https://doi.org/10.1007/978-3-0348-0439-4_10

6. Klambauer, G., Unterthiner, T., Mayr, A., Hochreiter, S.: Self-normalizing neural networks. In: Advances in Neural Information Processing Systems, pp. 971–980 (2017)

7. Browne, C.B., et al.: A survey of monte carlo tree search methods. IEEE Trans. Comput. Intell. AI Games **4**, 1–43 (2012)

8. Nguyen, D., et al.: Dose prediction with U-net: a feasibility study for predicting dose distributions from contours using deep learning on prostate IMRT patients. arXiv preprint arXiv:1709.09233 (2017)

Feasibility of CT-Only 3D Dose Prediction for VMAT Prostate Plans Using Deep Learning

Siri Willems[1]([✉]), Wouter Crijns[2], Edmond Sterpin[2,3], Karin Haustermans[2], and Frederik Maes[1]

[1] Department of ESAT, Processing Speech and Images (PSI), and UZ Leuven, Medical Imaging Research Center, KU Leuven, 3000 Leuven, Belgium
siri.willems@kuleuven.be
[2] Department of Oncology,
Laboratory of Experimental Radiotherapy, and UZ Leuven, Radiation Oncology, KU Leuven, 3000 Leuven, Belgium
[3] Department of Radiation Oncology, Cliniques uniersitaires Saint-Luc, UC Louvain, 1200 Woluwe-Saint-Lambert, Belgium

Abstract. Current radiotherapy planning workflows start with segmentation of the organs at risk (OARs) together with target volumes (TVs) in order to determine a patient specific optimal treatment plan and its corresponding 3D dose distribution. This is a time-consuming optimization process including many manual interventions. Despite strong resemblance between patients treated for the same indication, the optimization is almost always performed without 3D prior knowledge. Automated segmentation of OARs and TVs and automated generation of dose distributions are thus expected to be more time-efficient. We investigate the feasibility of CT-only dose prediction and the profitability of additional isocenter and contour information. To evaluate the network's performance, a 5-fold cross-validation is performed on 79 prostate patients, all treated with volumetric modulated arc therapy.

Keywords: Dose prediction · Isocenter · Convolutional neural networks

1 Introduction

Radiotherapy (RT) is one of the main treatments for prostate cancer, which relies on a patient specific treatment plan to deliver the prescribed radiation dose to the target volume (TV), while minimizing the dose to the healthy tissue, i.e. the organs at risk (OARs). Three main target volumes are defined in RT. The gross tumour volume (GTV) is the tumour and extent of the tumour visible on diagnostic images. The clinical target volume includes the GTV with an extra margin for subclinical disease spread which is not fully visible on medical images.

© Springer Nature Switzerland AG 2019
D. Nguyen et al. (Eds.): AIRT 2019, LNCS 11850, pp. 10–17, 2019.
https://doi.org/10.1007/978-3-030-32486-5_2

Lastly, the planning target volume (PTV) adds a margin to the CTV to account for uncertainties during treatment delivery.

Last decades, overall plan quality has improved, caused by recent evolution in RT planning, such as intensity modulated radiotherapy (IMRT) and volumetric modulated arc radiotherapy (VMAT) [1,2]. Apart from quality benefits, these treatment modalities enlarge planning time, hereby hampering the clinical implementation of adaptive strategies, which proved to have a positive effect on tumor control probability and post treatment complications [3–5].

The current RT planning workflow starts with the delineation of the TV and OARs. Next a complex inverse optimization procedure including a prior set of dose constraints identifies the optimal machine parameters required to administer the appropriate dose to the TVs and OARs [6]. This semi-automatic optimization process requires multiple adjustments of dose constraints and their priorities in order to assure convergence towards an optimal treatment plan. However, the manual interventions introduce interplanner variability, which may result in suboptimal solutions [7].

Recently, the research focus of RT has shifted towards knowledge based planning strategies, which utilize historical patient information to more efficiently generate RT treatment plans for newly diagnosed patients. More specifically deep learning by convolutional neural networks (CNNs) has been applied successfully in RT for segmentation tasks [8,9] and also for voxelwise dose prediction [10–13], assuming availability of contours and learning the contour-dose relationship.

These CNNs are very successful but the impact of the different inputs is not fully understood, e.g. the contours are implicitly present in the CT image. In this work we explore the impact of the contours by comparing dose prediction with and without contours as input. Additionally the potential impact of the, in classic treatment planning, crucial information of the isocenter is compared with the above scenarios.

2   Methods

2.1   Available Data and Preprocessing

The dataset consists of 79 patients diagnosed with prostate cancer [14]. All patients were treated with VMAT, receiving a prescription dose of 77 Gy fractionated over 35 treatment sessions, with 36 patients receiving a simultaneously integrated boost (SIB). The planning CT image of each patient was made on a multidetector-row spiral CT scanner (Somatom Sensation Open, 40 slice configuration; Siemens Medical Solutions, Erlangen, Germany). Segmentations of OAR and TV were performed manually by an experienced radiation oncologist and radiologist. The patient specific treatment plans and corresponding 3D dose distributions were created in clinical practice using Eclipse (Varian Medical Systems, Palo Alto, CA) and delivered with Clinac 2100C/D or TrueBeam (STx) (Varian Medical Systems, Palo Alto, CA).

The planning CT image is resampled to a voxelsize of $(2.5 \times 2.5 \times 3)\,\text{mm}^3$ and normalised to have zero mean and a standard deviation equal to 1. Dose distributions were normalised such that the mean dose within the PTV is equal to one. A GTV mask is created to distinguish SIB and standard procedures and contains the GTV delineation multiplied with a value of 95 if a SIB of 95 Gy is delivered to the patient's tumor and 0 if otherwise. Additional spatial context is derived from the 3D position of the isocenter, i.e. the center of rotation of the treatment gantry, located inside the prostate. For each voxel in the CT image, the X, Y and Z coordinates with respect to the isocenter are calculated. This results in 3 image grids for each CT image, containing either X, Y or Z coordinates w.r.t. the isocenter that we provided to the network.

2.2   Model Architectures

The baseline network architecture (CT-only model) is based on UNET and contains 4 pathways, see Fig. 1 [15]. Each pathway consist of 2 convolutional layers followed by batch normalization and a parametric linear rectified unit (PRELU) as non linear activation layer. Moreover each pathway contains extra residual connections. The final layer is a linear layer to predict the dose value such that the output represents a 3D dose distribution. The second model (CT+ISO) receives isocenter information by concatenating additional X, Y and Z image grids to the network after the upsampling part of UNET. Both the CT-only and CT+ISO model contain only the CT image and a GTV mask to indicate receival of a SIB as input. The third network (CT+C) and the fourth network (CT+ISO+C) are similar to the CT-only and the CT+ISO model resp., but are given all contours as extra input features to evaluate the effect of contours on voxelwise dose prediction.

2.3   Sampling and Training

Training is performed using a 3D patch-based approach and samples of size (156, 156, 78) are taken from the CT image using a weighted sampler. 50% of the samples are taken from the high dose region (i.e. dose greater than 80% of the prescription dose), 25% from the penumbra (i.e. dose between 20% and 80% of the prescription dose) and 25% from the low dose region (i.e. dose lower than 20% of the prescription dose), to ensure all dose regions are present during training. Adam optimizer is used for training with mean squared error as loss function.

2.4   Validation Experiment

A 5-fold cross-validation is performed in order to asses the influence of the isocenter information for CT-only dose prediction. These CT-only dose predictions are further compared to models using contour information as input. The predicted dose distributions of all four models (CT-only, CT+ISO, CT+C and CT+ISO+C) are compared using the clinical dose constraints (dmax, d98, d50, d2), derived from the dose volume histograms, which relate tissue volumes with

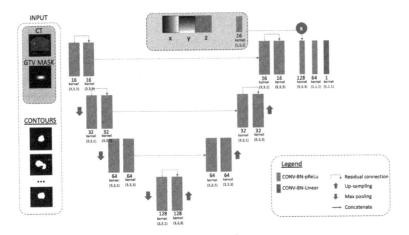

Fig. 1. 3D UNET architecture for dose prediction using either CT, CT+ISO, CT+C or CT+ISO+C as input features.

irradiated dose. The percentage error on these dose constraints relative to the prescription dose is calculated as follows for each structure:

$$\%\Delta DC_i = 100 * |\frac{f(\hat{D}_i) - f(D_{T,i})}{D_{pr,i}}| \tag{1}$$

with f equal to the dose constraint (dmax, d99, d98, d50 or d2), $\hat{D}_i$ and $D_{T,i}$ representing the predicted dose resp. the ground truth dose in organ i for a specific patient. $D_{pr,i}$ defines the prescription dose for the organ of interest more specifically 95 Gy for the SIB, and 77 Gy for all other organs.

Moreover the average dose volume histograms are established for all models for the PTV using the available ground truth contours.

3   Results

The cross-validation results for the target volumes (SIB, PTV, CTV) for all clinical indices are summarized in Table 1 for both the results before and after normalization as a post processing step, which is a well known step within RT for treatment plan optimization. The dose distribution is than multiplied with a constant such that the mean dose within the PTV equals the prescription dose. Overall the dose for the standard cases is better predicted than the dose for the SIB cases before normalization. The CT+ISO model outperforms the CT-only model on all clinical indices for both standard cases and the SIB cases. The lowest error rates are observed for dmax, d2 and d50, while higher error rates for d98 indicate lower dose conformity to the target volumes. The CT+C model and the CT+ISO+C model show decreased error rates for d98 towards both models without contour information, leading to a more conform dose distribution

Table 1. Error rate on clinical dose indices for the target volumes before and after dose normalization: PTV, CTV and SIB. Statistical significant differences are defined using pairwise wilcoxon test with $\alpha = 0.05$. Significant differences between the models with and without isocenter are indicated in bold fonts. Significant differences between models with and without contours are indicated with *.

Before Normalization		STAND				SIB			
		Dmax	D_2	D_{50}	D_{98}	Dmax	D_2	D_{50}	D_{98}
CT-only	SIB					15.7±6.4			
	PTV	6.3±3.2*	7.4±2.8*	11.7±2.5*	26.5±11.6	18.5±6.8	13.7±4.7	12.7±4.1	25.1±12.5
	CTV	6.3±3.2*	7.0±3.1*	10.5±2.6*	19.0±9.1	18.5±6.8	14.7±5.1	11.3±4.1	19.6±10.5
CT+ISO	SIB					7.2±4.8			
	PTV	**3.0±1.8**	**3.1±1.9**	**5.7±2.9**	21.1±15.9	**8.7±5.4**	**5.7±3.4**	**6.0±2.8**	**18.3±10.9**
	CTV	**2.8±1.6**	**2.9±1.7**	**4.1±2.6**	12.3±11.1	**8.8±5.4**	**6.6±3.7**	**4.8±2.5**	**12.8±9.3**
CT+C	SIB					14.7±5.1			
	PTV	13.4±3.0	13.4±2.6	13.6±2.5	12.3±3.0*	18.8±5.4	16.2±3.2	13.4±2.9	12.4±3.8*
	CTV	13.1±3.0	13.1±2.7	13.4±2.6	11.9±2.8*	18.8±5.4	17.0±3.6	13.2±3.0	12.4±5.1*
CT+ISO+C	SIB					4.8±4.0*			
	PTV	**1.6±1.3**	**1.5±0.9***	**1.8±1.1***	**3.2±2.0***	**6.8±4.0***	**3.6±2.2***	**2.0±1.7***	**2.9±2.3***
	CTV	**1.7±1.3**	**1.5±1.1**	**1.6±0.9***	**1.3±1.2***	**6.9±4.0***	**4.5±2.3***	**1.7±1.7***	**1.9±2.1***

After Normalization		STAND				SIB			
		Dmax	D_2	D_{50}	D_{98}	Dmax	D_2	D_{50}	D_{98}
CT-only	SIB					6.1 ±5.2			
	PTV	8.6±4.5	6.8±3.5	1.5±1.3	16.8±11.5	6.5±6.1	4.4±4.4	1.8±1.5	14.2±12.7
	CTV	8.7±4.5	7.2±3.5	2.9±2.0	7.9±8.2	6.6±6.1	4.7±4.4	3.6±2.2	7.3±9.9
CT+ISO	SIB					4.9±5.1			
	PTV	**6.2±3.4**	5.6±3.1	1.6±1.9	16.2±15.3	5.8±3.2	4.0±2.9	1.4±4.0	12.6±11.7
	CTV	**6.7±3.3**	6.2±3.1	3.3±2.4	6.4±9.4	5.9±5.9	4.6±4.6	3.0±1.7	6.5±7.9
CT+C	SIB					5.3±4.0			
	PTV	1.3±1.3*	0.7±0.7*	0.3±0.2*	1.0±2.4*	6.1±4.3	3.0±2.2*	0.5±0.5*	1.6±2.0*
	CTV	1.4±1.6*	1.0±1.1*	0.4±0.3*	1.4±1.2*	6.1±4.4	3.9±2.6*	0.8±0.8*	2.3±3.5*
CT+ISO+C	SIB					4.1±4.4			
	PTV	2.5±1.2*	2.0±0.8*	0.7±0.3*	1.6±2.7*	5.3±4.5	2.6±2.1*	**0.6±0.6***	1.3±1.3*
	CTV	2.9±1.3*	2.6±0.9*	1.2±0.5*	1.5±1.4*	5.5±4.4	3.2±2.3*	1.1±0.8*	1.6±1.3*

without a steep dose fall off at the border of the PTV. The best results are observed for the CT+ISO+C model on all clinical indices for both the standard and the SIB cases.

Normalization of the predicted dose distribution outcome of the CT-only, CT+ISO and CT+ISO+C models slightly increase the error on the Dmax, while the error of d50 decreases for the standard prostate cases. The error rates for the CT+model are decreased drastically after post processing the outcomes. For the SIB cases on the other hand, almost all error rates are improved compared to no post processing.

The error rate on the maximum dose (dmax) is visualised in Fig. 2(A) for both target volumes and OAR. The error rates are mainly negative, which indicates that all models show some lower dose estimation than the ground truth dose distributions created in Eclipse. Figure 2(B) shows the error rate on the maximum dose after normalization of all output dose predictions such that the mean dose within the PTV is equal to the prescription dose. Normalization of

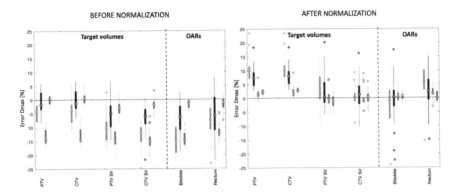

Fig. 2. Dmax error rate with respect to the prescription dose for standard cases for the initial dose prediction (A) and normalised output prediction (B). CT-only (pink), CT+ISO (blue), CT+C (green), CT+ISO+C (red) (Color figure online)

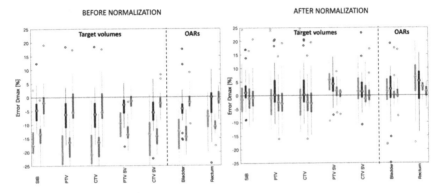

Fig. 3. Dmax error rate with respect to the prescription dose for SIB cases for the initial dose prediction (A) and normalised output prediction (B). CT-only (pink), CT+ISO (blue), CT+C (green), CT+ISO+C (red) (Color figure online)

dose distributions leads to higher dose to the target volume, but hereto results in positive error rates for the OAR compared to the ground truth dose distribution, which may exceeds the limiting dose constraint. The same trend is observed for the SIB cases, see Fig. 3. The best results are observed for the CT+ISO+C model before and after normalization, which slightly overstimates the target volumes, but preserves a lower dose to the OAR, i.e. bladder and rectum. The average dose volume histogram of the PTV over all patients for all previous discussed situations are visualised in Fig. 4.

4 Discussion

We evaluated the impact of the different inputs for dose prediction including isocenter and contour information. CT-only dose prediction including isocenter

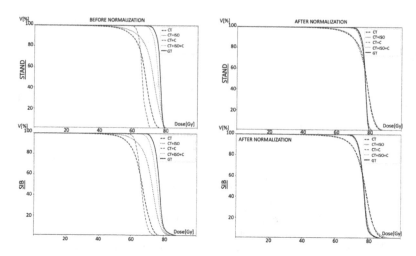

Fig. 4. Average Dose volume histograms (DVHs) for the PTV for all models before and after normalization for both standard cases (left) and SIB cases (right)

information outperforms the model without isocenter information and achieves reasonable results regarding maximum (Dmax) and median dose (d50) values. However, both models learn a relationship from CT hounsfield units to dose gray values without ever being forced to use the anatomy present in the CT image due to the mean squared error loss function. While the CT-only model underestimates the dose distribution for the TVs and OAR, isocenter information improves the results slightly by enlarging spatial information in the form of position restrictions. However a low d98 is observed which could be either due to a low dose conformity or low dose homogeneity of the PTV. Normalization of these dose distributions increases the dose in general but would still result in cold and hot spots around the target volume, hereby increasing the error on the maximum dose.

Providing contours as prior information, results in an overall better dose conformity and dose homogeneity, while minimizing the overestimation of dose to the OARs. The reason hereto is that the network receives anatomy information from the beginning. Furthermore, normalization of the output dose distribution has more benefits in this case, due to the higher conformity and homogeneity of the dose distributions. Adding isocenter information additionally to contour information, less dose normalization is necessary in order to obtain a good dose distribution. Moreover the obtained results for the model using isocenter and contour information are similar to those described in literature [10].

To be able to administer this dose in clinical practice, a treatment plan containing the optimal machine parameters should be established using a tool called 'dose mimicking'. To define the overall benefits of the isocenter and contour information, dose mimicking itself should be taken into account in future studies.

5   Conclusion

We demonstrate that isocenter information has a dose normalization effect, while contour information remains important to obtain more homogeneous dose distributions. Dose mimicking is necessary to define treatment parameters, which may in turn also influence the final dose slightly.

References

1. Craft, D.L., et al.: Improved planning time and plan quality through multicriteria optimization for intensity-modulated radio-therapy. Int. J. Radiat. Oncol. Biol. Phys. **82**(1), 83–90 (2012)
2. Otto, K., et al.: Volumetric modulated arc therapy: IMRT in a single gantry arc. Med. Phys. **35**(1), 310–317 (2007)
3. Nijkamp, J., et al.: Adaptive radiotherapy for prostate cancer using kilovoltage cone-beam computed tomography: first clinical results. Int. J. Radiat. Oncol. Biol. Phys. **70**(1), 75–82 (2008)
4. Yan, D., et al.: Adaptive radiation therapy. Phys. Med. Biol. **42**(1), 123–132 (1997)
5. Yand, H., et al.: Replanning during intensity modulated radiation therapy improved quality of life in patients with nasopharyngeal carcinoma. Int. J. Radiat. Oncol. Biol. Phys. **85**(1), 47–54 (2013)
6. Oelfke, U., et al.: Intensity modulation, inverse planning, proton-therapy, radiation therapy. Med. Dosim. **26**(2), 113–124 (2001)
7. Nelms, B., et al.: Variation in external beam treatment plan quality: an inter-institutional study of planners and planning systems. Pract. Radiat. Oncol. **2**(4), 296–305 (2012)
8. Ibragimov, B., et al.: Segmentation of organs-at-risks in head and neck CT images using convolutional neural networks. Med. Phys. **44**(2), 547–557 (2017)
9. Van der Veen, J., Willems, S., et al.: Benefits of deep learning for delineation of organs at risk in head and neck cancer. Radiother. Oncol. **138**, 68–74 (2019)
10. Nguyen, D., et al.: Dose prediction with U-net: a feasibility study for predicting dose distributions from contours using deep learning on prostate IMRT patients. Arxiv (2017)
11. Nguyen, D., et al.: Three-dimensional radiotherapy dose prediction on head and neck cancer patients with a hierarchically densely connected U-net deep learning architecture. Arxiv (2018)
12. Fan, J., et al.: Automatic treatment planning based on 3D dose distribution predicted from deep learning technique. Med. Phys. **46**(1), 370–381 (2018)
13. Kearney, V., et al.: A volumetric dose prediction algorithm using 3D fully- convolutional neural networks. Phys. Med. Biol. **63**(23), 61–78 (2018)
14. Lips, I.M., et al.: Single blind randomized phase III trial to investigate the benefit of a focal lesion ablative microboost in prostate cancer (FLAME-trial): study protocol for a randomized controlled trial (2011)
15. Ronneberger, O., Fischer, P., Brox, T.: U-Net: convolutional networks for biomedical image segmentation. In: Navab, N., Hornegger, J., Wells, W.M., Frangi, A.F. (eds.) MICCAI 2015. LNCS, vol. 9351, pp. 234–241. Springer, Cham (2015). https://doi.org/10.1007/978-3-319-24574-4_28

Automatically Tracking and Detecting Significant Nodal Mass Shrinkage During Head-and-Neck Radiation Treatment Using Image Saliency

Yu-chi Hu[1]([⊠]), Cynthia Polvorosa[2], Chiaojung Jillian Tsai[1], and Margie Hunt[1]

[1] Memorial Sloan Kettering Cancer Center, New York, NY 10065, USA
huj@mskcc.org
[2] Northern Westchester Hospital, 400 East Main Street, Mt Kisco, NY 10549, USA

Abstract. Large nodal masses shrink during head-and-neck radiation treatment. If the shrinkage is dramatic, nearby organs at risk (OARs) may receive potentially harmful radiation dose. In an institutional IRB-approved protocol, patients were monitored with weekly T2-weighted MRIs. Gross tumor volumes (GTV) from pre-treatment MRI were propagated to weekly MRIs via deformable image registrations (DIR) for tracking the change of GTV nodal volume and detection of significant shrinkage. This detection method, however, becomes problematic when a significant amount of the nodal mass dissolves during treatment, invalidating the assumption of correspondence between images for accurate deformable registration. We presented a novel method using image saliency to detect whether a involved nodal volume becomes significantly small during the treatment. We adapted a multi-resolution pyramid method and introduced symmetry in calculating image saliency of MRI images. The ratio of mean saliency value (RSal) from the propagated nodal volume on a weekly image to the mean saliency value of the pre-treatment nodal volume was calculated to assess whether the nodal volume shrank significantly. We evaluated our method using 94 MRI scans from 19 patients enrolled in the protocol. We achieved AUC of 0.97 in detection of significant shrinkage (smaller than 30% of the original volume) and the optimal RSal is 0.698.

Keywords: Image saliency · Nodal tumor shrinkage · Radiotherapy · Adaptive Radiation Therapy (ART)

1 Introduction

1.1 Clinical Background

Radiation therapy (RT) is one of the main treatment options for head-and-neck (H&N) cancer patients. The most common type of radiation therapy is called external-beam radiation (XRT) in which high-energy rays (or beams) are

© Springer Nature Switzerland AG 2019
D. Nguyen et al. (Eds.): AIRT 2019, LNCS 11850, pp. 18–25, 2019.
https://doi.org/10.1007/978-3-030-32486-5_3

delivered by a linear accelerator to deposit radiation dose from outside the body into the tumor.

A specific type of external-beam radiation therapy is intensity-modulated radiation therapy (IMRT) which uses advanced technology to modify the radiation beam to match the precise contour of a gross tumor volume (GTV) and minimize the damage to surrounding normal organs at risk (OARs). To achieve this, a treatment plan is generated using a computed tomography (CT) scan acquired prior to treatment delivery. The CT scan allows the team to capture patient specific anatomical geometry for beam optimization and precise dose calculations. The plan, however, does not consider potential changes to the patients' anatomy during a treatment course. Therefore, the results of the dose distribution may deviate from initial plan during treatment. Occasionally, large GTV nodal volumes demonstrate dramatic shrinkage [1,2] during 5–7 week treatment course. With IMRT, the dosimetric consequences of such changes could be significant, particularly when the target is adjacent to critical OARs. Our observations show that critical structures may move into sharp high dose areas created in the original treatment plan. Adaptive radiotherpay (ART) [3,5,6] aims to observe the anatomical changes during the treatment using repeating imaging during treatment and adjust the initial plan accordingly.

1.2 Monitoring Volume Changes Using Deformable Image Registration

Deformable image registration (DIR) has been widely used to automatically propagate regions of interests (ROIs) from pre-treatment images to the most recent images to identify anatomical deviations during a radiotherapy course. For simplicity, Eq. 1 shows the cost function commonly used in DIR algorithms to be minimized for obtaining a displacement vector field v.

$$C(v) = S(I_{fixed}, v(I_{moving})) + R(v) \tag{1}$$

S is a similarity term that penalizes differences between a fixed image I_{fixed} and the deformed moving image $v(I_{moving})$. R is a regularization term to control smoothness of the displacement vector field.

Studies have shown that while DIR performed well for OARs, DIR-propagated GTVs still require expert correction [4]. In our study, although we used T2-weighted MRI images for superior soft tissue contrast compared to CT, the average Dice score for propagated nodal volumes dropped from 0.85 at week 1 to 0.72 at week 4. For the similarity term to work in DIR algorithms, the tissue must exists on both fixed and moving images. Such assumption becomes invalid at certain stages within the treatment course due to tissue loss, a resultant of significant tumor regression. Figure 1 shows an example of substantial nodal tumor regression. A majority of cancerous tissues visible on the pre-treatment T2 MRI image disappeared on week 4 image taken during the treatment. The nodal volume propagated from pre-treatment image to week 4 image could no longer accurately detect the significant volume shrinkage.

We propose a novel approach that analyzes salient regions of images along with DIR-propagated volumes to accurately and automatically detect significant tumor regression during the treatment to facilitate adaptive radiotherapy.

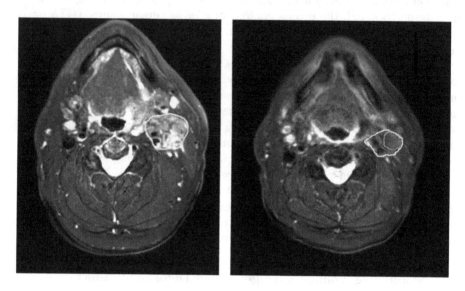

Fig. 1. The nodal volume (red) on the pre-treament T2-weighted MRI image (left) was propagated to the week 4 image (right) which does not agree well with the ground truth drawn by a physician (cyan). (Color figure online)

2   Methods

2.1   Image Saliency

On H&N T2-weighted MRI images, nodal GTVs often exhibit distinct perceptual quality which makes tumor tissue visually emerge from neighboring normal tissues and attract our attention. Visual attention regions can be automatically identified using an image saliency map. Figure 2 shows our proposed framework to generate an image saliency map from an image by adapting a classic method [7]. An intensity Gaussian pyramid is first generated from MRI images. We then applied Gabor filters at 0, 45, 90 and 135° to generate orientation features at each scale of the intensity Gaussian pyramid. In addition, we introduced a symmetry feature to highlight locations of the abnormal tissue. In H&N cancer, malignancies often spread to lymph nodes on one side of the neck depending on the location from which the primary tumor originated. In contrast, normal H&N images are symmetrical. We define the symmetry feature as a point-wise subtraction:

$$Sym(Y) = |Y - Flip_{LR}(Y)|, \tag{2}$$

where $Flip_{LR}(Y)$ is the horizontally flipped image of Y in left-right direction. Figure 2 shows our proposed framework to generate an image saliency map.

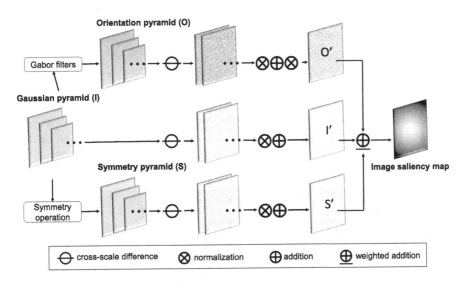

Fig. 2. Image saliency framework.

For each feature pyramid (intensity, orientation and symmetry), across-scale difference, denoted "$\ominus$", between a finer scale $s \in \{2, 3, 4\}$ and a coarser scale $c = s + \delta, \delta \in \{3, 4\}$ was calculated by interpolation to the finer scale and point-wise subtraction:

$$\ominus I(s, c) = |I(s) - I_{\uparrow s}(c)|, \tag{3}$$

$$\ominus S(s, c) = |S(s) - S_{\uparrow s}(c)|, \tag{4}$$

$$\ominus O(s, c, \theta) = |O(s, \theta) - O_{\uparrow s}(c, \theta)|, \tag{5}$$

where I, S, O are the feature maps for intensity, symmetry and orientation respectively, $\uparrow s$ is interpolation to scale s, and θ is the degree of Gabor filter.

The resulting cross-scale difference maps then were normalized to eliminate amplitude differences between feature maps and to elevate maps in which a small number of strong peaks of activity stand out, while underplaying maps containing numerous peaks that have similar activities. Given a map x, the normalization operator $\otimes$ is defined as

$$\otimes x(i) = (1 - \overline{m}_w(x_{[0...1]}, i))^2 x_{[0...1]}(i), \tag{6}$$

where $x_{[0...1]}$ is the map normalized to range $[0...1]$ and $\overline{m}_w$ is the mean of local maximums given a local window size w. The normalized cross-scale feature maps are then resized and united to generate an feature-specific attention map using point-wise addition.

$$I' = \oplus_{s \in \{2,3,4\}, c=s+\delta, \delta \in \{3,4\}}^{\uparrow 1} \otimes (\ominus I(s, c)), \tag{7}$$

$$S' = \oplus_{s\in\{2,3,4\},c=s+\delta,\delta\in\{3,4\}}^{\uparrow1} \otimes (\ominus S(s,c)), \tag{8}$$

$$O' = \sum_{\theta\in\{0°,45°,90°,135°\}} \otimes(\oplus_{s\in\{2,3,4\},c=s+\theta,\theta\in\{3,4\}}^{\uparrow1} \otimes (\ominus O(s,c,\theta))), \tag{9}$$

The final saliency map is created from a linear and weighted combination of the feature-specific attention maps:

$$Sal(x) = \oplus(I'_x, S'_x, O'_x) = w_I I'_x + w_S S'_x + w_O O'_x, \tag{10}$$

Figure 3 shows the image saliency maps corresponding to Fig. 1. The involved nodal volume (depicted by the arrow) shows high saliency in the map of the pre-treatment image (left), comparing to low saliency at the same location on the week 4 image (right) acquired during the treatment as the tumor regressed.

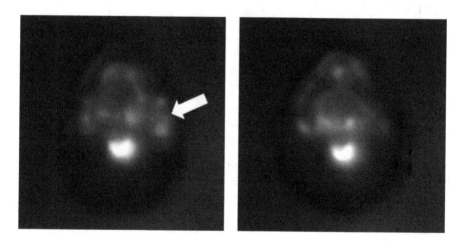

Fig. 3. The image saliency maps corresponding to Fig. 1.

2.2   Detection Metric for Significant Nodal Volume Shrinkage

While DIR may lose track of volumes should there be significant nodal volume shrinkage during treatment as discussed in Sect. 1. The incorrectly deformed volumes could still be useful in detecting significant volume shrinkage by analyzing image information inside the deformed volumes. Given a nodal target structure $NGTV$ defined in the pre-treatment image Y_{pre}, we define a ratio of saliency metric (RSal) as

$$RSal(NGTV, t) = \overline{Sal}_{x, x\in NGTV_t}(Y_t)/\overline{Sal}_{x, x\in NGTV}(Y_{pre}), \tag{11}$$

where $NGTV_t$ be the DIR-propagated volume on the image Y_t acquired at time point t during the treatment, and $\overline{Sal}_x$ is the mean saliency value of voxels inside the structure.

The idea of using a ratio is that the node's un-treated volume and regressed volume attract different attention levels. When the shrinkage is extensive, the location where the original nodal volume was located (identified by $NGTV_t$), is most certainly occupied by normal tissues and fluid, therefore, should attract much less attention compared to the original nodal target ($NGTV$).

3 Experiments

3.1 Data Set

Our experiment data set included 94 pre-treatment and weekly T2-weighted fat-suppression MRI image series from 19 patients recruited on an institutional IRB-approved protocol. Pre-treatment nodal target volumes were manually delineated by physicians and were approved for treatment planning. In addition, weekly nodal volumes were manually delineated by physicians or senior planners and served as ground truth to quantify nodal GTV shrinkage.

3.2 Volume Propagation

A DIR algorithm developed by MIM Software^{TM} (Beachwood, OH) was used for deformable image registrations between pre-treatment and weekly images. Pre-treatment volumes were propagated onto weekly images by applying the displacement fields from DIR. The process was fully automated without human intervention.

3.3 Evaluation

Studies [1,2] reported a mean relative shrinkage of nodal GTV to be 45–50% after 20 treatment days. We evaluated our method (**RSal**) in the detection of significant shrinkage: whether the weekly volume of nodal GTV is (1) smaller than 40% and (2) smaller than 30% of the initial volume. For comparison, we used shrinkage calculated from DIR-propagated volumes (**Xform**) as the control. In addition, we randomly sampled 5000 points inside each nodal GTV in the pre-treatment images and transformed the points to weekly images using the displacement vectors from DIR. We then calculated the normalized cross-correlation (**NCC**) of the intensities from the sample points in the pre-treatment image and transformed sample points in the weekly images as another metric in the comparisons. We used ROC (receiver operating characteristic) for performance measurement for the detection accuracy.

3.4 Results

In detecting volume of nodal GTV that is smaller than 40% of the initial volume, Area under ROC curve (AUC) for RSal, NCC and XForm are 0.89, 0.85 and 0.86 respectively. RSal achieved specificity of 0.83 and sensitivity of 0.84 using the optimal threshold 0.799. In detecting volume of nodal GTV that is smaller than 30% of the initial volume, AUC for RSal, NCC and XForm are 0.97, 0.93 and 0.83 respectively. RSal achieved specificity of 0.92 and sensitivity of 0.90 using the optimal threshold 0.698. Figures 4 and 5 show the ROC plots of performance comparison in detecting significant shrinkage.

In terms of computation time, the saliency calculation is within 40 ms for a 256 × 256 MRI slice.

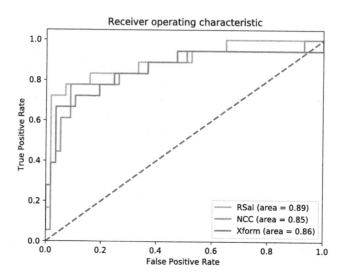

Fig. 4. ROC plot of performance in detecting the volume of nodal GTV smaller than 40% of the initial volume.

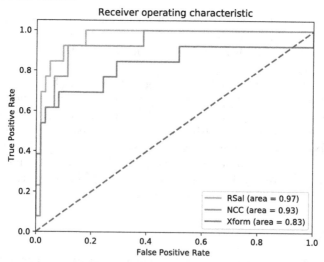

Fig. 5. ROC plot of performance in detecting the volume of nodal GTV smaller than 30% of the initial volume.

4   Conclusion and Future Works

Tracking and detecting significant nodal volume shrinkage during the radiation treatment can facilitate adaptive planning to avert potentially harmful dose to nearby OARs. We propose a novel approach using image saliency to detect significant volume shrinkage and introduced a symmetry feature in saliency calculation. The experiment results showed that our method can achieve high accuracy in detection and is computationally inexpensive. We are currently increasing our patient cohort, evaluating such patient cases for further investigation. In particular, we are looking at the dosimetric modifications resulting from GTV nodal volume change to help develop a trigger that can alert physicians when a volume change is significant enough to warrant the need for plan adaptation.

References

1. Sanguineti, G., et al.: Volumetric change of human papillomavirus-related neck lymph nodes before, during, and shortly after intensity-modulated radiation therapy. Head Neck **34**, 1640–1647 (2012). https://doi.org/10.1002/hed.21981
2. Castadot, P., Lee, J.A., Geets, X., Grégoire, V.: Adaptive radiotherapy of head and neck cancer. Semin. Radiat. Oncol. **20**(2), 84–93 (2010). https://doi.org/10.1016/j.semradonc.2009.11.002
3. Hansen, E.K., Bucci, M.K., Quivey, J.M., Weinberg, V., Xia, P.: Repeat CT imaging and replanning during the course of IMRT for head-and-neck cancer. Int. J. Radiat. Oncol. Biol. Phys. **64**(2), 355–363 (2006). https://doi.org/10.1016/j.ijrobp.2005.07.957
4. Hardcastle, N., Tomé, W.A., Cannon, D.M., et al.: A multi-institution evaluation of deformable image registration algorithms for automatic organ delineation in adaptive head and neck radiotherapy. Radiat. Oncol. **7**(1), 90–96 (2012). https://doi.org/10.1186/1748-717X-7-90
5. Woodford, C., Yartsev, S., Dar, A.R., Bauman, G., Van Dyk, J.: Adaptive radiotherapy planning on decreasing gross tumor volumes as seen on megavoltage computed tomography images. Int. J. Radiat. Oncol. Biol. Phys. **69**, 1316–1322 (2007). https://doi.org/10.1016/j.ijrobp.2007.07.2369
6. Wu, Q., Chi, Y., Chen, P.Y., Krauss, D.J., Yan, D., Martinez, A.: Adaptive replanning strategies accounting for shrinkage in head and neck IMRT. Int. J. Radiat. Oncol. Biol. Phys. **75**, 924–932 (2009). https://doi.org/10.1016/j.ijrobp.2009.04.047
7. Itti, L., Koch, C., Niebur, E.: A model of saliency-based visual attention for rapid scene analysis. IEEE Trans. PAMI **20**(11), 1254–1259 (1998). https://doi.org/10.1109/34.730558

4D-CT Deformable Image Registration Using an Unsupervised Deep Convolutional Neural Network

Yang Lei, Yabo Fu, Joseph Harms, Tonghe Wang, Walter J. Curran,
Tian Liu, Kristin Higgins, and Xiaofeng Yang[✉]

Department of Radiation Oncology and Winship Cancer Institute,
Emory University, Atlanta, GA 30322, USA
xiaofeng.yang@emory.edu

Abstract. Four-dimensional computed tomography (4D-CT) has been used in radiation therapy to allow for tumor and organ motion tracking throughout the breathing cycle. It can provide valuable information on the shapes and trajectories of tumor and normal structures to guide treatment planning and improve the accuracy of tumor delineation. Respiration-induced abdominal tissue motion causes significant problems in effective irradiation of abdominal cancer patients. Accurate and fast deformable image registration (DIR) on 4D-CT could aid the treatment planning process in target definition, tumor tracking, organ-at-risk (OAR) sparing, and respiratory gating. However, traditional DIR methods such as optical flow and demons are iterative and generally slow especially for large 4D-CT datasets. In this paper, we present our preliminary results on using a fast-unsupervised generative adversarial network (GAN) to generate deformation vector fields (DVF) for 4D-CT DIR to help motion management and treatment planning in radiation therapy. The proposed network was trained in an unsupervised fashion without the need of ground truth DVF or anatomical labels. A dilated inception module (DIM) was integrated into the network to extract multi-scale motion features for robust feature learning. The network was trained and tested on 15 patients' 4D-CT abdominal datasets using five-fold out cross validation. The experimental results demonstrated that the proposed method could attain an accurate DIR between any two 4D-CT phases within one minute.

Keywords: 4D-CT · Image registration · Unsupervised deep learning

1 Introduction

Respiration-induced abdominal tissue motion causes significant problems in treatment planning and radiation delivery for abdominal cancer patients. 4D-CT has been used in radiation therapy for treatment planning to reduce dose to healthy organs and increase dose to the tumor target [1, 2]. Deformable image registration (DIR) could be used to process the 4D-CT images and track internal organ movement. Accurate and fast DIR on 4D-CT could facilitate multiple treatment planning processes such as target definition, tumor tracking, OAR sparing and respiratory gating. However, traditional DIRs [3] such as optical flow and demons are iterative and generally very slow especially for

© Springer Nature Switzerland AG 2019
D. Nguyen et al. (Eds.): AIRT 2019, LNCS 11850, pp. 26–33, 2019.
https://doi.org/10.1007/978-3-030-32486-5_4

large 4D-CT datasets. Therefore, it is necessary to develop a fast and accurate for 4D-CT DIR to aid motion management and treatment planning process in radiation therapy.

Deep learning-based image registration methods can be divided into three categories: deep iterative registration, supervised transformation estimation, and unsupervised transformation estimation [4]. Deep iterative registration algorithms aim to augment the performance of traditional, iterative, intensity-based registration methods by using deep similarity metrics. Therefore, deep iterative registration algorithms have the same limitation of slow processing speed as the traditional registration algorithms. Supervised transformation estimation algorithms utilize either manually aligned image pairs in the case of full supervision or manually defined anatomical structure labels in the case of weak supervision. Manual preparation of large sets of training datasets is laborious, subjective and error-prone. To avoid manual processes, synthetic images can be generated by deforming the fixed image with an artificial DVF for the supervision of the transformation estimation networks. However, the artificial DVF may lead to biased training since the artificial DVF is unrealistic and can be very different from physiological motion.

In this paper, we focused on unsupervised deep learning DIR methods. Ghosal et al. proposed another unsupervised DIR for 3D MR brain images by optimizing the upper bound of the sum of squared difference (SSD) between the fixed image and the deformed image [5]. Their method outperformed the log-demons based registration. An unsupervised feature selection framework for 7T MR brain images was proposed by Wu et al. using a convolutional-stacked autoencoder network [6]. However, this method still inherits the existing iterative optimization for DVF calculations, which is computation slow. De Vos et al. trained a fully convolutional neural network (FCN) using normalized cross correlation (NCC) to perform 4D cardiac cine-MR volume registration [7]. They showed that their method has outperformed Elastix based registration [8]. These unsupervised methods were mainly focused on 2D/3D MR brain images and cardiac images. Compared to MR brain images registration, abdominal 4D-CT image registration is more challenging due to the poorer image contrast and significant abdominal motion in 4D-CT. The large respiration-induced abdominal motion poses additional difficulties in image registration and DVF regularization. To overcome these challenges, we have developed a novel unsupervised generative adversarial network (GAN)-based method to directly estimate the DVF from any two phases of abdominal 4D-CT images in a single forward prediction. A dilated inception module (DIM) was integrated into the network generator to extract multi-scale structural features for robust feature learning. Nonlinear sparse regularization was used to enforce sparseness of DVF within the small-motion or static regions. The gradient and bending energy of the predicted DVF were penalized to ensure the smoothness and physical fidelity of the deformation field.

2   Methods

Section 2.1 provides a system overview of the proposed DIR model and the preprocessing steps to prepare training datasets. In Sect. 2.2, we detail the network architecture of the proposed model. The network losses and DIR regularizations are described in Sect. 2.3.

2.1   4D-CT Training and Testing Data and System Overview

We trained our 4D-CT DIR model using data from a clinical database of 15 patients undergoing radiation therapy. For each patient, the dataset contains 10 CT images, which are binned according to the breathing cycle, that were acquired using a Siemens CT scanner. The resolutions of the 4D-CT datasets range from $0.9 \times 0.9 \times 2.5$ mm to $1.2 \times 1.2 \times 2.5$ mm depending on the patient size. The proposed DIR model was designed to perform DIR between any two phases of a 4D-CT dataset. The proposed network was trained and tested using five-fold cross-validation.

Figure 1 illustrates our method's model training and DIR workflow. Our model was designed in a 3D patch-based fashion. The training data were collected via extracting pairs of 3D patches from the moving and fixed images by sliding a window of $48 \times 48 \times 64$ voxels. To enlarge the variety of training data, the overlap size between two neighboring patches was set to $24 \times 24 \times 32$ voxels, and any two different phases of each training patient were regarded as moving and fixed CT images. The patch size in the superior-inferior direction was set to be 64 instead of 48 since the respiration-induced abdominal motion was larger in this direction than the other two directions.

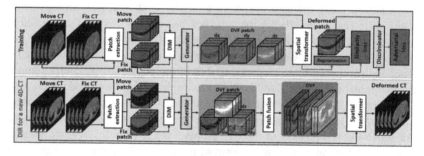

Fig. 1. The schematic flow diagram of the proposed method. The upper row shows the training stage for DVF inference. The lower row shows the DIR procedure where one phase was deformed to match another phase in a new 4D-CT.

The motion information of a pair of moving and fixed patches was first coarsely learned by a DIM. Then, it was fed into a generator to learn deeper features and to map to an equal sized DVF. The deformed patch was obtained by registering the moving patch via a spatial transformer with DVF. To optimize the DIM and the generator, both the regularization of DVF and the performance of generated DVF for registration were taken into account. For unsupervised training, additional regularization is necessary due to the lack of a ground truth DVF. Therefore, we incorporated an adversarial loss term in the optimization to avoid unrealistic DVF prediction.

After training the model, a DVF between any two phases of a new patient was obtained by feeding the moving and fixed patches into the trained model to estimate DVF patches, then fusing the DVF patches together to whole image's DVF. The moving phase was deformed to fixed phase using the whole-image DVF.

2.2   Network Architecture

The proposed network has three separate sub-networks with a DIM and generator dedicated for DVF inference and a discriminator dedicated to judge how realistic a deformed patch looks. Figure 2 shows the architectures of these three sub-networks.

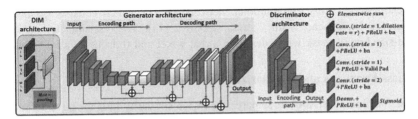

Fig. 2. The architecture of proposed GANs including one generator and one discriminator.

The proposed DIM was inspired by Google's Inception Module (GIM) [9] which consists of three convolutional kernels of different sizes and a same sized max-pooling, The module attempts to compare and capture motion information from different scales for later DVF estimation. However, the number of trainable parameters increases significantly as the convolutional kernel size increases [10]. To reduce the computational cost, we proposed a dilated convolution with fixed kernel size and different dilation rates in this study. Compared to GIM, the proposed dilated inception module can achieve the same receptive field as that of the GIM with much fewer trainable parameters. The dilated convolutional kernels with different dilation rates can extract multi-scale information from the images [11]. 4D-CT provides high in-plane resolution images with abundant information which require extensive computational resources without yielding much benefit. The dilated convolutional kernels are more efficient than the common inception module in skipping the redundant voxel-by-voxel information and extracting only the representative multi-scale textures. We reported the number of trainable parameters needed to achieve the same reception field for both the dilated inception module and the common inception module in Table 1. For comparison, the common inception module needs 31.8 times more parameters than the dilated inception module to achieve same receptive filed.

The generator was implemented in an end-to-end U-Net fashion [12]. Residual blocks [13], which aimed to learn the structural differences between the moving and fixed patches, were used for the skip connections between same sized feature maps extracted from encoding and decoding paths in generator.

Table 1. Comparison of the number of trainable parameters needed to achieve same reception field between GIM and DIM.

	Layers	Kernel size	# Feature maps	# Parameters	Total
GIM	Conv1	$6 \times 6 \times 6$	8	1736	21408
	Conv2	$9 \times 9 \times 9$	8	5840	
	Conv3	$12 \times 12 \times 12$	8	13832	
DIM	Conv1 r = 2	$3 \times 3 \times 3$	8	224	672
	Conv2 r = 3	$3 \times 3 \times 3$	8	224	
	Conv3 r = 4	$3 \times 3 \times 3$	8	224	

The discriminator is used to judge the realism of the deformed patch against the fixed patch. As shown in the discriminator architecture, the discriminator is a typical classification-based fully convolutional network (FCN), which consists of multiple convolutional layers, each with a stride size of 2 [14]. The discriminator outputs a reduced-size binary mask with 1 denoting a real voxel and 0 denoting a fake voxel.

2.3 Loss Functions and Regularizations

The loss function consists of three parts: the image similarity loss, the adversarial loss, and the regularization loss.

$$
G = \underset{G}{\arg\min} \left\{ \begin{array}{c} 1 - CC\left(I^{\circ}_{mov}\varphi, I_{fix}\right) + \alpha \cdot GD\left(I^{\circ}_{mov}\varphi, I_{fix}\right) \\ + \beta \cdot ADV\left(I^{\circ}_{mov}\varphi, I_{fix}\right) + \gamma \cdot R(\varphi) \end{array} \right\} \tag{1}
$$

where $\varphi = G\left(I_{mov}, I_{fix}\right)$ represents the predicted deformation field for a fix and moving image patch pair. The deformed image patch, $I^{\circ}_{mov}\varphi$, was obtained by warping the moving image patch by the predicted deformation field using a spatial transformation. $CC(\cdot)$ denotes the cross-correlation loss, $GD(\cdot)$ denotes the gradient difference loss between the fix and moving image patches. The cross-correlation loss and gradient loss of the images together represent the image similarity loss. $ADV(\cdot)$ denotes the adversarial loss, which is computed as the discriminator cross entropy loss of the deformed and fixed patches after central cropping. The central cropping was utilized to avoid boundary effects during registration. The cropped image patch size was $36 \times 36 \times 48$. The discriminator is implemented using a conventional FCN. The purpose of the adversarial loss was to encourage the deformed image to look like a realistic image by penalizing implausible DVFs and unreasonably deformed images. $R(\varphi)$ denotes the regularization term.

$$
R(\varphi) = \|\varphi\|_2 + \mu_1 \|\nabla\varphi\|_2 + \mu_2 \|\nabla^2\varphi\|_2 \tag{2}
$$

The proposed regularization term includes weighted terms of a l_2-norm of the predicted DVF and its first and second derivatives. The l_2-norms of the first and second derivatives of DVF were used to enforce general smoothness of the predicted DVF. We observed that the motion between any two phases of 4D-CT are very small for most of the background region. Therefore, we aimed to enforce the sparsity of the predicted DVF to register regions with minor motion. Adam gradient optimizer with learning rate of 1e−5 was used for optimization.

3 Results

Five-fold cross-validation testing was performed on 15 4D-CT abdominal patients' datasets. We randomly partitioned the 15 patients 4D-CT images into five equal sized subgroups. One subgroup was retained as the validation data for testing the model, and the remaining four subgroups were used as the training data. Mean absolute error (MAE), peak signal-to-noise ratio (PSNR) and normalized cross correlation (NCC) were calculated between the deformed and fixed images for quantitative evaluations. At least three fiducial markers were placed inside patient for pancreas tumor localization. Target registration errors (TREs) were calculated based on these fiducial markers for the proposed method.

Figure 3 shows a comparison of the proposed method with and without DIM. Part of the images shown in (b3) look unrealistic, suggesting an inaccurate deformation field around this region. In comparison, the image in (b5) shows significant improvement over (b3), indicating the importance of the dilated inception module. The comparison between (b4) and (b6) also suggests that using the dilated inception module could largely improve the registration accuracy. Similar phenomena were observed on the sagittal views, i.e. (d3–d6) and coronal views i.e. (f3–f6).

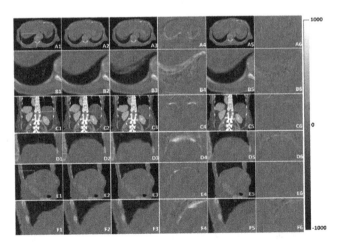

Fig. 3. Comparison between results computed with and without DIM. Images from left to right are the moving, fixed, deformed image without using DIM, difference image between the deformed image without using DIM and fixed image, deformed image using DIM, and the difference image between the deformed image using DIM and the fixed image.

Figure 4 shows an example of deformed CT image from moving image to fixed (reference) image. This deformed CT is close to fixed CT images. Table 2 shows the numerical results between the deformed and fixed CT for each patient. Overall, the mean MAE, PSNR, NCC and TRE were 15.6 ± 4.6 HU, 38.0 ± 3.3 dB, 0.996 ± 0.002 and 2.48 ± 0.98 mm, which demonstrated the deformation accuracy of the proposed method.

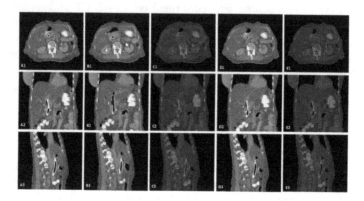

Fig. 4. 4D CT registration results. Images from left to right are the fixed, moving and fusion image between the fixed and moving images before registration, deformed images, fusion image between the fixed and deformed images after registration.

Table 2. Numerical evaluation of the proposed method.

	MAE (HU)	PSNR (dB)	NCC	TRE
Proposed	15.6 ± 4.6	38.0 ± 3.3	0.996 ± 0.002	2.48 ± 0.98

4   Conclusion and Discussion

The method proposed can be used for lung and abdominal 4D-CT DIR, which in turn can be used as a promising tool for lung and abdominal motion management and treatment planning during radiation therapy. The proposed method allows accurate DIR between any two 4D-CT phases within one minute. For this preliminary study, we used cross correlation and gradient difference as image similarity loss function to optimize the network. Other image similarity metrics such as mean absolute error and mutual information could be used together with the cross correlation to improve the performance. Since the network was trained in an unsupervised manner without any prior knowledge about the correct physiological motion patterns, the DVF regularization was especially important for accurate DVF predictions. In this study, only spatial smoothness and DVF sparsity were used for regularization, which might not be sufficient. The DVF sparsity constraint worked well in regions where motion was minimal, i.e. the bone. It does not work very well in regions where both poor image contrast and large motion are present, i.e. within the liver. Future work will incorporate prior DVF knowledge to the regularization.

Acknowledgements. This research is supported in part by the National Cancer Institute of the National Institutes of Health under Award Number R01CA215718, and Dunwoody Golf Club Prostate Cancer Research Award, a philanthropic award provided by the Winship Cancer Institute of Emory University.

Disclosure. The authors declare no conflicts of interest.

References

1. D'Souza, W.D., et al.: The use of gated and 4D CT imaging in planning for stereotactic body radiation therapy. Med. Dosim. **32**(2), 92–101 (2007)
2. Tai, A., Liang, Z., Erickson, B., Li, X.: Management of respiration-induced motion with 4-dimensional computed tomography (4DCT) for pancreas irradiation. Int. J. Radiat. Oncol. **86**(5), 908–913 (2013)
3. Yang, X., et al.: Automated segmentation of the parotid gland based on atlas registration and machine learning: a longitudinal MRI study in head-and-neck radiation therapy. Int. J. Radiat. Oncol. **90**(5), 1225–1233 (2014)
4. Haskins, G., Kruger, U., Yan, P.: Deep learning in medical image registration: a survey. ArXiv, abs/1903.02026 (2019)
5. Ghosal, S., Rayl, N.: Deep deformable registration: enhancing accuracy by fully convolutional neural net. Pattern Recogn. Lett. **94**, 81–86 (2017)
6. Wu, G., Kim, M., Wang, Q., Munsell, B.C., Shen, D.: Scalable high-performance image registration framework by unsupervised deep feature representations learning. IEEE Trans. Bio-Med. Eng. **63**(7), 1505–1516 (2016)
7. de Vos, B.D., Berendsen, F.F., Viergever, M.A., Staring, M., Išgum, I.: End-to-end unsupervised deformable image registration with a convolutional neural network. In: Cardoso, M.J., et al. (eds.) DLMIA/ML-CDS -2017. LNCS, vol. 10553, pp. 204–212. Springer, Cham (2017). https://doi.org/10.1007/978-3-319-67558-9_24
8. Klein, S., Staring, M., Murphy, K., Viergever, M.A., Pluim, J.P.W.: Elastix: a toolbox for intensity-based medical image registration. IEEE Trans. Med. Imaging **29**(1), 196–205 (2010)
9. Szegedy, C., et al.: Going deeper with convolutions. In: IEEE CVPR 2015, pp. 1–9 (2015)
10. Wang, B., et al.: Deeply supervised 3D fully convolutional networks with group dilated convolution for automatic MRI prostate segmentation. Med. Phys. **46**(4), 1707–1718 (2019)
11. Zhu, H.C., et al.: Dilated dense U-net for infant hippocampus subfield segmentation. Front. Neuroinform. **13**, 30 (2019)
12. Ronneberger, O., Fischer, P., Brox, T.: U-net: convolutional networks for biomedical image segmentation. In: Navab, N., Hornegger, J., Wells, W.M., Frangi, A.F. (eds.) MICCAI 2015. LNCS, vol. 9351, pp. 234–241. Springer, Cham (2015). https://doi.org/10.1007/978-3-319-24574-4_28
13. Gao, F., Wu, T., Chu, X., Yoon, H., Xu, Y., Patel, B.: Deep residual inception encoder-decoder network for medical imaging synthesis. IEEE J. Biomed. Health Inform. (2019, in press)
14. Lei, Y., et al.: MRI-only based synthetic CT generation using dense cycle consistent generative adversarial networks. Med. Phys. **46**(8), 3565–3581 (2019)

Toward Markerless Image-Guided Radiotherapy Using Deep Learning for Prostate Cancer

Wei Zhao, Bin Han, Yong Yang, Mark Buyyounouski, Steven L. Hancock, Hilary Bagshaw, and Lei Xing$^{(\boxtimes)}$

Stanford University, Stanford, CA 94306, USA
{zhaow85,hanbin,yongy66,mbuyyou,shancock,hbagshaw,lei}@stanford.edu

Abstract. Current image-guided prostate radiotherapy often relies on the use of implanted fiducial markers (FMs) or transducers for target localization. Fiducial or transducer insertion requires an invasive procedure that adds cost and risks for bleeding, infection and discomfort to some patients. We are developing a novel markerless prostate localization strategy using a pre-trained deep learning model to interpret routine projection kV X-ray images without the need for daily cone-beam computed tomography (CBCT). A deep learning model was first trained by using one thousand annotated projection X-ray images. The trained model is capable of identifying the location of the prostate target for a given input X-ray projection image. To assess the accuracy of the approach, six patients with prostate cancer received volumetric modulated arc therapy (VMAT) were retrospectively studied. The results obtained by using the deep learning model and the actual position of the prostate were compared quantitatively. Differences between the predicted target positions using DNN and their actual positions are (mean ± standard deviation) 1.66 ± 0.41 mm, 1.63 ± 0.48 mm, and 1.64 ± 0.28 mm in anterior-posterior, lateral, and oblique directions, respectively. Target position provided by the deep learning model for the kV images acquired using OBI is found to be consistent that derived from the implanted FMs. This study demonstrates, for the first time, that highly accurate markerless prostate localization based on deep learning is achievable. The strategy provides a clinically valuable solution to daily patient positioning and real-time target tracking for image-guided radiotherapy (IGRT) and interventions.

Keywords: Image-guided radiation therapy · Deep learning · Markerless tracking

1 Introduction

Radiotherapy is an effective, targeted therapy for the management of clinically-localized prostate cancer, which accounts for over 28% of total cancer cases in the United States. Recent advance of highly conformal external-beam radiotherapy,

D. Nguyen et al. (Eds.): AIRT 2019, LNCS 11850, pp. 34–42, 2019.
https://doi.org/10.1007/978-3-030-32486-5_5

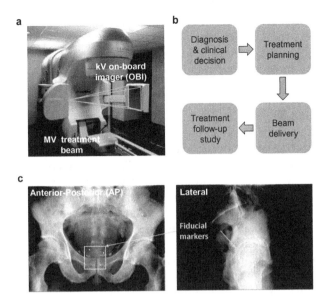

Fig. 1. External-beam radiotherapy. a. Clinical radiation treatment machine with imaging guidance using on-board flat-detector imager. b. Pipeline of radiotherapy. c. Implanted gold fiducial markers used for daily positioning and real-time tracking in image-guided radiotherapy.

such as volumetric modulated arc therapy (VMAT), has greatly augmented our ability to shape the toxicity profile by conforming radiation dose to the tumor target while sparing the normal tissue. However, just being able to produce conformal dose distributions is not enough as it only fulfills part of the requirements of precision radiotherapy. This is because the position of prostate may change from both inter-fraction and intra-fraction motion. For patients to truly benefit from the advanced planning and dose delivery techniques, we must also ensure that the planned dose is delivered to the right location and at the right time [5,7,15]. Hence, an effective imaging method for real-time tumor localization is very important for precision radiotherapy.

However, there are limited real-time image guidance strategies for radiotherapy. The recently developed and released on-board magnetic resonance imaging (MRI) technique requires huge amount of hardware support and cost [1], which poses a significant burden for most radiotherapy treatment sites. Intra-fraction monitoring using ultrasound is possible, but its tracking accuracy is inferior and thus it is still at early stage of development [10]. Instead, the use of stereoscopic or monoscopic kV X-ray imaging with on-board imager (Fig. 1a) amounted on the most of the currently available radiotherapy facilities can provide high accuracy and it is more practicable [15]. While using this method, the low prostate contrast makes it difficult to see the prostate on the projection X-ray images. Thus, metallic fiducial markers (FMs) are often implanted into the prostate to facilitate the patient setup and real-time tumor tracking [3,13], as shown in Fig. 1c. However, the implantation of the FM is an invasive procedure which may introduce bleeding, infection and discomfort to the patient. It also requires the service of an interventional radiologist or other specialist and prolongs the treatment procedure. Besides, studies have shown FM can migrate within the patient and the prostate exhibits random deformation leading to uncertainty to target localization [9].

As a part of machine learning, deep learning has been leveraged in the whole radiotherapy pipeline except beam delivery, which includes tumor diagnosis and staging [2], treatment planning [6,16], and follow up studies [4], as shown in Fig. 1b. However, no prior efforts have been devoted to the key component, beam delivery. Here, we report the development and validation of a patient-specific deep-learning model, based on a realistic training data generation scheme, to achieve marker-free location of treatment target for prostate IGRT. We validate the localization accuracy using independent validation datasets on orthogonal directions to show the feasibility of daily positioning, and an oblique direction to show the feasibility of real-time tracking. Validation using positioning kV images acquired with OBI is also included. We believe this is a major step forwards for deep learning in IGRT and is essential for fully machine intelligence powered external-beam radiotherapy.

2   Materials and Methods

2.1   Deep Learning for Tumor Target Localization

The workflow of the proposed deep learning-based target localization process for prostate IGRT include three steps. The first step is to generate training datasets of kV projection X-ray images reflecting various situations of the anatomy, including different level of rotation, organ deformation, and translation of the patient. For this purpose, robust deformable models described by motion vector fields (MVFs) are used to deform simulation CT to different clinical scenarios. The second step is to generate digitally reconstructed radiographs (DRR) for each deformed CT dataset in a predefined direction. Finally, the annotated samples are used to train a deep learning model for subsequent localization of the prostate target. Validation tests using both simulated DRR and clinical on-board imager (OBI) daily positioning images were performed. More details are described in the following subsections.

2.2   Generation of Labeled Training Datasets for Deep Learning

Due to the low contrast of the prostate, we propose to generate kV projection images for different anatomical positioning scenarios from augmented pCT for a specific patient. In order to obtain the labeled DRR images which incorporate numerous possible clinical statuses (such as positioning and shapes) of the involved anatomical structures to train the deep learning model for a specific patient at specific direction, a well validated deformable image registration method [14] is employed to extract the general MVFs which are used to deform the planning CT data. The deformations are performed together with other possible transformations (rotation and random translation) in clinical scenarios. Specifically, for the pCT images of each patient, we first introduce rotations (from $-4°$ to $4°$ with $2°$ interval) to the images around superior-interior direction. Then, to deform the high-quality planning CT data, we extract MVFs by registering pre-treatment daily positioning cone-beam CT (CBCT) data from different courses of treatment with respect to the well-defined pCT. After applying the MVFs to the rotation incorporated pCT images, a series of 250 CT data that cover different clinical scenarios are generated and these data are used to mimic the specific patient in different positions and statuses. The deformed CT datasets are then divided into two parts, where 225 deformed CT datasets are used for model training and the other 25 deformed CT datasets are used for model testing.

The corresponding DRRs along the directions of anterior-posterior (AP), left-right (LR), and oblique degree ($135°$) are then generated for each deformed CT data using accurate X-ray reprojection model. In the reprojection calculation, we use the realistic OBI geometry with the source to detector distance of 1500 mm and the source to patient distance of 1000 mm. The projection pixel size and array size are the same as the OBI. The DRR calculation is implemented using CUDA C with graphics processing unit (Nvidia GeForce GTX Titan X, Santa Clara, CA) acceleration. Each of the DRR is then randomly shifted 4 times to further increase the sample sizes. Hence, a total of 900 DRRs are generated for each projection direction for the training of deep learning model for the specific patient, and 100 DRRs are used for testing. To annotate the DRRs, for each patient, we extract the delineated prostate contour used for treatment planning. The prostate is applied to the same changes (deformations, rotations, translations) as the pCT data. The prostate after change is reprojected using consistent OBI geometry to produce prostate-only projection for the corresponding simulated kV projection. The bounding box of the prostate for the prostate-only projection is then calculated and is regarded as an annotation of the corresponding simulated kV image (DRR). The DRRs and the corresponding bounding box information (top-left corner, width, height) are used to train a deep learning model.

2.3 Deep Learning Model

With the annotated datasets, we are able to train a deep learning model to localize the prostate for IGRT without implanted FMs. In our deep learning model, the input is either a DRR image or a monoscopic X-ray projection image

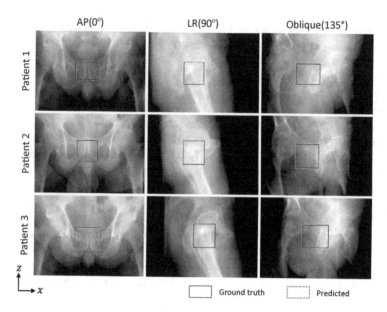

Fig. 2. Examples of the prostate boundary boxes derived from the deep learning model (yellow dashed box) and their corresponding annotations (blue box), overlaid on top of the patients DRRs. The first, second and third columns show the results in AP, oblique and L-Lat directions, respectively. In all directions, the predicted prostate position agrees with the known position better than 3 mm. (Color figure online)

acquired by the OBI system from a given direction, and the output is the location of the treatment target. In this study, we train a faster-rcnn model to localize the prostate. The model includes a region-proposed network and a region-based convolutional neural network and these two networks can share the feature hierarchies to achieve real-time detection [12]. Hence, it is desirable for target tracking in radiotherapy. We use VGG16 ConvNet as the feature extractor and 10 epochs to train the network. The learning rate is set to 0.001. For efficient training of the deep learning model, the annotated samples are cropped into the size of 700 × 1000. Before training, all training samples are randomly permuted.

2.4   Validation of the Prostate Localization Model

In this institutional review board-approved HIPPA-compliance study, the deep learning-based prostate localization model is validated by retrospective analysis of 6 VMAT patients. Patients have a median age of 77 (range, 70–85). For each patient, the pCT images along with the structure file for treatment planning and patient setup images (CBCT images or orthogonal kV fiducial images) were retrieved from Varian External Beam Planing system (Eclipse, Varian Medical System, Palo Alto, CA). A set of 900 synthetic DRRs was generated for each of

Table 1. Mean absolute difference and Lin's concordance correlation coefficients between the predicted and annotated prostate positions in anterior-posterior, left-right, and oblique directions. Data are shown as means ± standard deviations.

Patient index		Anterior-posterior		Left-lateral		Oblique	
		Deviations (mm)	ρ_c	Deviations (mm)	ρ_c	Deviations (mm)	ρ_c
1	Δx	1.78 ± 1.77	0.95	2.16 ± 1.43	0.93	1.63 ± 1.26	0.96
	Δz	0.98 ± 0.64	0.97	1.15 ± 0.78	0.92	1.28 ± 0.97	0.93
2	Δx	2.07 ± 1.22	0.96	1.50 ± 1.20	0.96	1.79 ± 1.22	0.95
	Δz	2.48 ± 2.32	0.91	1.19 ± 0.80	0.89	1.69 ± 1.05	0.91
3	Δx	1.50 ± 1.08	0.95	2.37 ± 1.70	0.93	1.50 ± 1.06	0.96
	Δz	1.82 ± 1.28	0.90	1.70 ± 0.71	0.91	1.36 ± 1.13	0.89
4	Δx	1.58 ± 1.10	0.97	2.51 ± 1.83	0.94	1.93 ± 1.65	0.96
	Δz	1.03 ± 0.69	0.93	1.49 ± 1.10	0.91	1.33 ± 0.93	0.93
5	Δx	1.78 ± 1.49	0.97	1.73 ± 1.28	0.96	2.16 ± 1.64	0.94
	Δz	1.45 ± 1.02	0.98	1.08 ± 0.78	0.94	1.81 ± 1.24	0.98
6	Δx	1.69 ± 1.51	0.96	1.48 ± 1.15	0.96	1.87 ± 1.86	0.97
	Δz	1.76 ± 1.58	0.94	1.27 ± 0.95	0.91	1.41 ± 1.31	0.94
Mean ± Std		1.66 ± 0.41		1.63 ± 0.48		1.64 ± 0.28	

three directions (AP, LR, and an oblique direction 135°) for each patient. These DRRs are employed to train a deep learning model, which was then tested using 100 independent DRRs. A patient whose prostate implanted FMs and was setup using the kV fiducial images acquired using OBI was also examined to directly show the potential of the method for prostate localization. Mean absolute difference (MAD) and Lin's concordance correlation coefficient (ρ_c) [8] was calculated to assess the results along with the difference between the annotated position and DNN predicted position of the prostate.

3 Results

Examples of the prostate bounding boxes (dashed yellow lines) predicted for three patients in AP, LR and oblique directions using the deep learning approach are shown in Fig. 2. Here the blue lines show the annotated bounding box obtained from the raw pCT images of the specific patients. It is seen clearly that the predicted bounding box positions match the annotated positions very well in all three directions for all patients. Table 1 summarizes the results of the Lin's concordance correlation coefficients and MADs between the model predicted positions and the annotated positions for all 6 patients. For all cases, the MADs are smaller than 3 mm and ρ_c values are greater than 0.89, suggesting the predicted positions and the annotated positions agree each other well.

Course 1   Course 2   Simulated projection

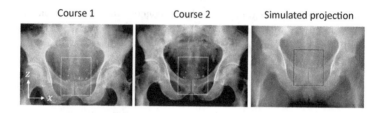

Fig. 3. Predicted and actual positions of the prostate target overlaid on top of the anterior-posterior simulated projections (3rd column) as well as the OBI images (1st and 2nd columns) for two different treatment courses of a patient who was setup using kV fiducial imaging. OBI = on-board imager.

It took about 2 h to train a specific model for a given direction for a patient. The training was performed on a server with configuration of Intel Core i7-6700K RAM 32 GB and Nvidia GeForce GTX Titan X GPU. Once the model is trained, it took less than 200 ms for prediction, which is very desirable for real-time tumor tracking during radiotherapy dose delivery, showing the merit of the proposed method.

Figure 3 shows the predicted prostate positions (the dashed yellow bounding box) in a simulated projection (DRR) and two kV fiducial images for two treatment courses. The kV fiducial images were acquired for daily positioning before the radiotherapy treatment. As can be seen, the predicted prostate position in the simulated projection is highly consistent with the annotated position, which is also consistent with the predicted positions in the kV fiducial images for the two courses. The patient has four implanted FMs and analysis of the positions of these markers relative to the corresponding bounding boxes afford additional assurance of the correctness of our deep learning model. In all these courses, the predicted prostate position is also found to be consistent with that indicated by the FMs, suggesting the proposed method can provide accurate prediction of prostate position for precision radiotherapy.

4   Summary

Normally, training a deep learning model require a large amount of annotated dataset which is very time-consuming for the data annotation. Hence, most of object detection algorithms, especially the newly developed algorithms are validated using public datasets which are well-annotated. While computer vision deal with existing natural images which are relatively easy to annotate, object detection in medical applications are mainly hindered by the data annotation, which requires well-trained clinicians and involves huge manpower, especially for the task in this study, i.e., X-ray imaging. Due to the low soft-tissue contrast, most of time, it is impossible to label the tumor target in the X-ray projection image without the implanted FMs, and deep learning-based tumor detection has only been applied to chest X-ray until now [11]. For other treatment sites, such as prostate, even a well-trained clinician can not identify the target.

This study is tackling the highly challenging problem by proposing a realistic training data generation scheme, which is then used to train a deep learning model for localization of prostate based on projection images acquired prior or during therapy for IGRT. The results on clinical prostate IGRT cases show the proposed approach can provide highly accurate prostate position. This is an attempt of applying deep learning to IGRT for the first time. Two novelties of the proposed approach are: (1) a realistic model training scheme by using the motion incorporated synthetic DRRs derived from the pCT images; and (2) a deep learning approach for nearly real-time localization of the prostate.

References

1. Acharya, S., Fischer-Valuck, B.W., Kashani, R., et al.: Online magnetic resonance image guided adaptive radiation therapy: first clinical applications. Int. J. Radiat. Oncol. Biol. Phys. **94**(2), 394–403 (2016)
2. Bejnordi, B.E., Veta, M., Van Diest, P.J., et al.: Diagnostic assessment of deep learning algorithms for detection of lymph node metastases in women with breast cancer. JAMA **318**(22), 2199–2210 (2017)
3. Campbell, W.G., Miften, M., Jones, B.L.: Automated target tracking in kilovoltage images using dynamic templates of fiducial marker clusters. Med. Phys. **44**(2), 364–374 (2017)
4. Cha, K., Hadjiiski, L., Chan, H., et al.: Bladder cancer treatment response assessment in CT using radiomics with deep-learning. Sci. Rep. **7**(1), 8738 (2017)
5. Cui, Y., Dy, J.G., Sharp, G.C., Alexander, B., Jiang, S.B.: Multiple template-based fluoroscopic tracking of lung tumor mass without implanted fiducial markers. Phys. Med. Biol. **52**(20), 6229 (2007)
6. Ibragimov, B., Xing, L.: Segmentation of organs-at-risks in head and neck CT images using convolutional neural networks. Med. Phys. **44**(2), 547–557 (2017)
7. Jaffray, D.A.: Image-guided radiotherapy: from current concept to future perspectives. Nat. Rev. Clin. Oncol. **9**(12), 688 (2012)
8. Lawrence, I., Lin, K.: A concordance correlation coefficient to evaluate reproducibility. Biometrics 255–268 (1989)
9. Nichol, A.M., Brock, K.K., Lockwood, G.A., et al.: A magnetic resonance imaging study of prostate deformation relative to implanted gold fiducial markers. Int. J. Radiat. Oncol.* Biol.* Phys. **67**(1), 48–56 (2007)
10. O'Shea, T., Bamber, J., Fontanarosa, D., et al.: Review of ultrasound image guidance in external beam radiotherapy part II: intra-fraction motion management and novel applications. Phys. Med. Biol. **61**(8), R90 (2016)
11. Rajpurkar, P., Irvin, J., Zhu, K., et al.: ChexNet: radiologist-level pneumonia detection on chest x-rays with deep learning. arXiv preprint arXiv:1711.05225 (2017)
12. Ren, S., He, K., Girshick, R., Sun, J.: Faster R-CNN: towards real-time object detection with region proposal networks. IEEE Trans. Pattern Anal. Mach. Intell. **6**, 1137–1149 (2017)
13. Shirato, H., Shimizu, S., Shimizu, T., Nishioka, T., Miyasaka, K.: Real-time tumour-tracking radiotherapy. Lancet **353**(9161), 1331–1332 (1999)

14. Vercauteren, T., Pennec, X., Perchant, A., Ayache, N.: Diffeomorphic demons: efficient non-parametric image registration. NeuroImage **45**(1), S61–S72 (2009)
15. Xing, L., Thorndyke, B., Schreibmann, E., et al.: Overview of image-guided radiation therapy. Med. Dosim. **31**(2), 91–112 (2006)
16. Zhen, X., Chen, J., Zhong, Z., et al.: Deep convolutional neural network with transfer learning for rectum toxicity prediction in cervical cancer radiotherapy: a feasibility study. Phys. Med. Biol. **62**(21), 8246 (2017)

A Two-Stage Approach for Automated Prostate Lesion Detection and Classification with Mask R-CNN and Weakly Supervised Deep Neural Network

Zhiyu Liu[1], Wenhao Jiang[1], Kit-Hang Lee[1], Yat-Long Lo[1],
Yui-Lun Ng[1], Qi Dou[2], Varut Vardhanabhuti[3],
and Ka-Wai Kwok[1(✉)]

[1] Department of Mechanical Engineering, The University of Hong Kong,
Pok Fu Lam, Hong Kong
kwokkw@hku.hk
[2] Department of Computing, Imperial College London, London, UK
[3] Department of Diagnostic Radiology, Li Ka Shing Faculty of Medicine,
The University of Hong Kong, Pok Fu Lam, Hong Kong

Abstract. Early diagnosis of prostate cancer is very crucial to reduce the mortality rate. Multi-parametric magnetic resonance imaging (MRI) can provide detailed visualization of prostate tissues and lesions. Their malignancy can be diagnosed before any necessary invasive approaches, such as needle biopsy, at the risk of damage to or inflammation of the periprostatic nerves, prostate and bladder neck. However, the prostate tissue malignancy on magnetic resonance (MR) images can also be difficult to determine, with often inconclusive results among the clinicians. With the progress in artificial intelligence (AI), research on MR image-based lesion classification with AI tools are being explored increasingly. So far, existing classification approaches heavily rely on manually labelling of lesion areas, which is a labor-intensive and time-consuming process. In this paper, we present a *novel* two-stage method for *fully-automated* prostate lesion detection and classification, using input sequences of T2-weighted images, apparent diffusion coefficient (ADC) maps and high b-value diffusion-weighted images. In the first stage, a Mask R-CNN model is trained to automatically segment prostate structures. In the second stage, a weakly supervised deep neural network is developed to detect and classify lesions in a *single* run. To validate the accuracy of our system, we tested our method on two datasets, one from the PROSTATEx Challenge and the other from our local cohort. Our method can achieve average area-under-the-curve (AUC) of 0.912 and 0.882 on the two datasets respectively. The proposed approach present a promising tool for radiologists in their clinical practices.

Keywords: Prostate cancer · MR images classification · Weakly supervised learning

© Springer Nature Switzerland AG 2019
D. Nguyen et al. (Eds.): AIRT 2019, LNCS 11850, pp. 43–51, 2019.
https://doi.org/10.1007/978-3-030-32486-5_6

1 Introduction

Prostate cancer is the second leading cancer-related cause of death in the male population [1], with the estimate that 1 in 9 men in the US will be diagnosed with prostate cancer in their lifetime [2]. The prostate-specific antigen (PSA) test is mainly used as an upfront screening test for men without symptoms. Men with PSA level >4 would have an increasing chance of prostate cancer, and will be followed-up by further tests, such as MRI. mpMRI is commonly employed before tissue biopsy. Diagnosis with MRI would reduce unnecessary biopsy by 70%. Daniel *et al.* [3] reported 486% increased use of mpMRI from Oct 2013 to Dec 2015. Thus, a lot of prostate magnetic resonance (MR) images require radiologists to interpret in current clinical routine. Recently, the Prostate Imaging Reporting and Data System [4] guidelines were established to standardize and minimize the variation in interpreting prostate MRI. Geoffrey *et al.* [5] observed variability in cancer yield across radiologists, with 24% of males who were assigned a score of having a benign lesion turned out to have clinically significant prostate cancer on biopsy. This false negative rate could vary from 13% to 60% among radiologists. With the advances of deep learning in medical imaging, our goal is to automate the diagnosis process by detecting and classifying prostate lesions with high accuracy in a single framework.

There have been several works on prostate lesion classification with multi-parametric MRI. Karimi *et al.* [6] proposed to combine hand-crafted features and learned features for classifying malignancy of prostate lesions mpMRI images, which led to an area-under-the-curve (AUC) of 0.87. Liu *et al.* [7] proposed XmasNet that reformulates 3D mpMRI images as a 2D problem. To incorporate 3D information when learning from 2D slices, they employed data augmentation through 3D rotation and slicing. The approach attained a performance of 0.84 AUC.

However, these methods require labeling of lesion centroid, which is necessarily done by clinicians. In a related research on prostate lesion detection and classification in MRI, Kiraly *et al.* [8] used a deep convolutional encoder-decoder architecture to simultaneously detect and classify prostate cancer, and they reached an average classification performance of 0.834 AUC. However, they applied a region of interest (ROI) of roughly the same size to ensure only the prostate and its surrounding areas were considered. Such simplification may lead to imprecision.

In this paper, we propose a novel two-stage framework for *fully*-automated prostate lesion detection and diagnosis. In the *first* stage, prostate zone/contour in MR images is automatically segmented. *Secondly*, an analytical framework is implemented to detect and classify malignancy of prostate lesions. The major work contributions are: (i) A Mask R-CNN [9] model is trained to segment/pinpoint a smaller ROI that contains all the lesion candidates. (ii) A weakly supervised deep neural network is developed to process the detection/classification in a *single* run. (iii) Detailed validation is conducted on two datasets, namely PROSTATEx Challenge [10] dataset and our local cohort. Classification performance is also compared with the state-of-the-art approaches.

2   Methods

Figure 1 illustrates our proposed two-stage automatic framework. We applied an object detection method, Mask R-CNN, to train a prostate segmentation model for T2-weighted images that show tissues in high contrast and brightness. The model outputs a smaller size image that contains the prostate ROI. With coordinate transformation, prostate regions in ADC maps and high *b*-value diffusion-weighted images become available. Next, the prostate ROI will act as input to a deep neural network (DNN), outputting lesion areas and classification results in one single feedforward pass. Malignancy of the classified lesions will then be determined through the ensemble learning of images of different input sequences.

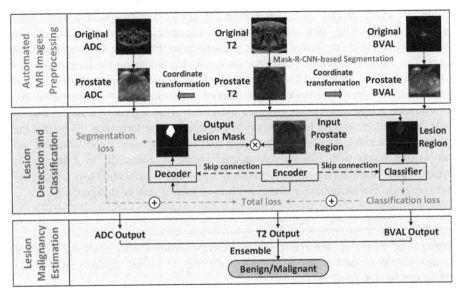

Fig. 1. Schematics of the proposed automated prostate lesion detection/classification.

2.1   Mask R-CNN for Automated Prostate Structures Segmentation

Prostate lesions detection can be difficult, as the lesions are small relative to the entire image size. Thus, identifying the prostate ROI is crucial to enable more accurate and effective lesion detection. Mask R-CNN object detection approach relies on generated region proposals, each of which outputs a class, bounding box, and a mask. Multi-scale features are extracted from various layers, which provide more powerful information to segment specific objects at various scales. These are particularly useful for our case, as the prostate sizes among patients can vary. To train this Mask R-CNN model, we employ an online prostate segmentation dataset, along with well labelled masks, which were released by the Initiative for Collaborative Computer Vision Benchmarking (I2CVB) [11]. The trained model can narrow the entire MR images down to the prostate ROI only, thus facilitating the subsequent detection and classification process.

2.2 Weakly Supervised Deep Neural Network for Prostate Lesion Detection and Classification

In the prostate classification datasets used by existing approaches, only lesion centroids are located, but not their exact outlines. Previous work [8] attempted to resolve this issue by applying lesion labels with identical gaussian distribution at each lesion point. However, this approach could not account for variations in lesion sizes. To this end, we employ a distance regularized level set evolution [12] to generate weak lesion labels. Provided with the lesion centroids, this method can be applied to edge-based active contour model for weak lesion labels.

Given the prostate region identified at stage one, we employed our novel weakly supervised DNN for simultaneous lesion detection and classification based on the weak masks and classification labels. The network comprises *three* key components, namely encoder, decoder and classifier. The encoder consists of five groups of convolutional layers and max-pooling layers while the decoder contains five upsampling layers. The encoder and decoder are linked with skip connections between their corresponding layers. The decoder is trained to produce lesion masks, indicating the location of predicted lesions. The predicted weak lesion mask, together with prostate region and features extracted from the encoder are then reused by the classifier. We hypothesize that the additional lesion and prostate structure masks can act as a form of attention map to guide the classifier, leading to the improved classification performance. To predict the malignancy of lesions, the classifier itself also contains five groups of convolutional and max-pooling layers with two fully connected layers. A composite loss function is applied, which combines the lesion segmentation loss and classification loss, to train the entire network. For each sample, the classification loss L_C can be designed as:

$$L_C = -y \log c(x) - (1-y) \log[1 - c(x)] \tag{1}$$

where $x \in \mathbb{R}^{w \times h}$, $y \in \mathbb{R}^1$ and $c(x) \in \mathbb{R}^1$, respectively, denotes input, label and output of the data sample; w and h are the width and height of input images. Lesion segmentation loss L_S can be described as:

$$L_S = 1 - \frac{2 \sum_i^w \sum_j^h \left[M_{i,j} S_{i,j}(x) \right] + \varepsilon}{\sum_i^w \sum_j^h M_{i,j} + \sum_i^w \sum_j^h S_{i,j}(x) + \varepsilon} \tag{2}$$

where, $M \in \mathbb{R}^{w \times h}$ and $S(x) \in \mathbb{R}^{w \times h}$, respectively, denote mask label and output mask of the lesion; $M_{i,j}$ and $S_{i,j}(x)$ represent pixel values of their corresponding masks in the i_{th} column and j_{th} row of matrix. The parameter ε is a numerical constant to avoid division of zero and ensure numerical stability. The total loss function L_T is also weighted with two coefficients, λ_C and λ_S as below. Note that the Adam [13] optimizer is applied to train the network with a learning rate of 10^{-6}.

$$L_T = \lambda_C L_C + \lambda_S L_S \tag{3}$$

3 Experimental Results

3.1 Prostate Structures Segmentation

In the *first* stage, 646 slices of T2-weighted images from 21 patients scanned with 1.5-T (GE) scanner and 15 patients scanned with 3.0-T (Siemens) scanner were extracted to train and validate our prostate segmentation model. We used a 7:2:1 split ratio for the slices extracted from the I2CVB dataset for training, validation and testing. Data augmentation was performed on the training sets by random rotation of [$\pm30°$, $\pm60°$, $\pm90°$]. All the inputs were resized to 512×512 pixels before feeding in the Mask R-CNN model. Learning rate is set to 10^{-3}. We trained on two GPUs with a batch size of 4 for 200 epochs. The model with the best dice coefficient on the validation set is chosen as final model, with results on the test split reported. Figure 2a shows a sample of segmentation result. As shown in Table 1, we have compared our results with other methods using mean intersection over union (IoU). These show that Mask R-CNN can achieve higher IoU in segmenting prostate and central gland. Our segmentation model can obtain prostate regions on T2 sequences of the two datasets (Fig. 2b and c).

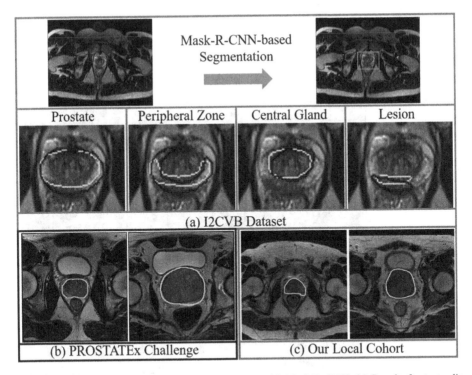

Fig. 2. Samples of automated prostate segmentation with Mask R-CNN. (a) Results for test split of I2CVB dataset. The ground truth is indicated in green, and the predicted area is in yellow. Predicted prostate area of PROSTATEx Challenge dataset (b) and our local cohort (c). (Color figure online)

3.2 Prostate Lesion Detection and Classification

In the *second* stage, our proposed weakly supervised network is trained and validated on PROSTATEx Challenge dataset (330 lesion samples, 76 malignant and 254 benign) and our local cohort (74 lesion samples, 51 malignant lesions and 23 benign lesions). We used GLEASON score (malignant for values ≥ 7) to label lesion malignancy on both datasets. We trained two sets of models on these two datasets. Each set of models consists of models trained on three sequences, namely T2-weighted images, ADC maps and high b-value diffusion-weighted images. All the segmented prostate regions were prepared for both datasets in stage one. Data augmentation was applied to the training data with random rotation of [$\pm 3°$, $\pm 6°$, $\pm 9°$, $\pm 12°$, $\pm 15°$]. The image sizes were then scaled to 224×224 pixels for training. We conducted 5-fold cross validation experiments on both datasets. Through repeated experimental trials, parameters weights λ_C and λ_S were both set to 1, with ε set to $10-5$. The final classification results and AUC were obtained through ensemble learning from all three sequences.

Table 1. Comparison of Mean IoU on I2CVB dataset with other methods.

Methods	Prostate	Central gland	Peripheral zone	Lesion
Ruba Alkadi - M1 [14]	–	0.673	0.563	0.677
Ruba Alkadi - M2 [14]	–	0.657	0.599	0.679
Mask R-CNN (ours)	**0.843**	**0.781**	0.516	0.405

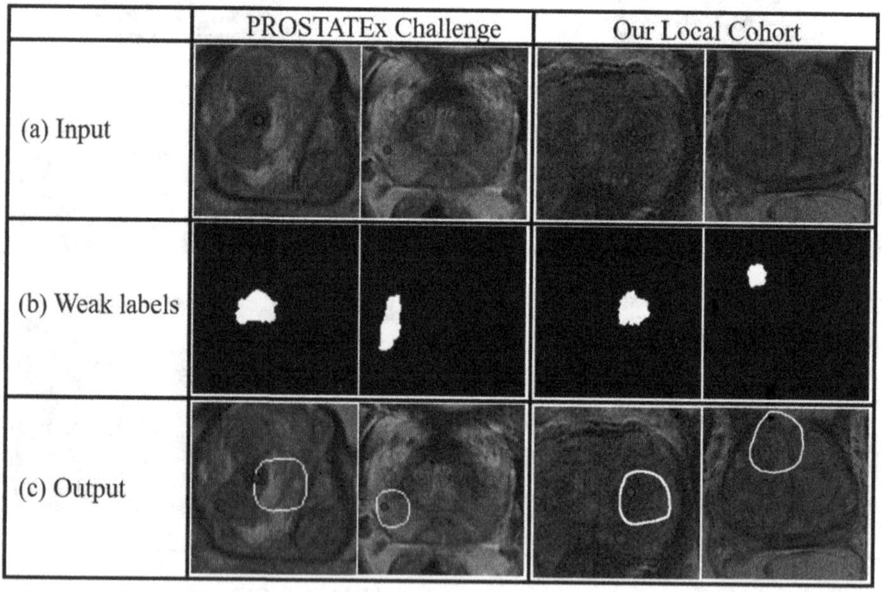

	PROSTATEx Challenge	Our Local Cohort
(a) Input		
(b) Weak labels		
(c) Output		

Fig. 3. Samples of result for lesion detection of T2-weighted images. Green spots indicate the given lesions centroid. (a) Input of raw prostate region. (b) Weak lesion mask obtained from level set method. (c) Predicted lesion area contoured by yellow. (Color figure online)

Figure 3 shows the results of lesion detection in T2 sequences. Figure 4a and b illustrate the final average receiver operating characteristic curve (ROC curve) on the two prostate lesion datasets with our proposed approach. For PROSTATEx Challenge dataset, our model outputs the average AUC of 0.912 with ensembled input sequences of ADC maps and T2-weighted images, outperforming the other two existing methods that individually combine hand-craft features and learned features (AUC of 0.870) [6], and encoder-decoder architecture (AUC of 0.834) [8]. For our local cohort, the average AUC of 0.882 is obtained with ensemble learning over input sequences. Moreover, we compare the results *without* pre-segmentation. Figure 4c and d indicate significantly *lower* AUC on the two datasets with the non-segmented/cropped image as input, showing the crucial role of pre-segmentation in this detection/classification framework.

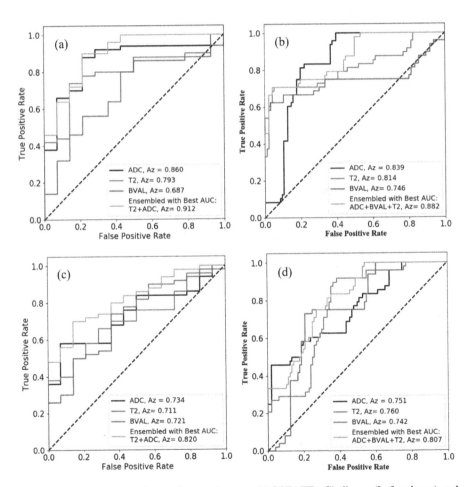

Fig. 4. Average AUC results on the two datasets: PROSTATEx Challenge (Left column) and our local cohort (Right column). AUC results (a) and (b) are input *with* prostate region segmented by Mask R-CNN models. Lower AUC can be observed in (c) and (d) *without* the segmentation.

4 Conclusion

This paper proposes a novel framework for *fully*-automated prostate lesion detection and diagnosis in MR images. Experiments on PROSTATEx Challenge dataset and our local cohort achieve a promising average AUC of 0.912 and 0.882 on their validation set respectively. The resultant efficacy is comparable to the first (champion) and second highest in AUC in PROSTATEx challenge [7], which achieved 0.87 and 0.84 on the test set, respectively. Our proposed method is extensible to other structures demanding for similar lesion diagnosis using MRI. For future work, we will extend the framework 3D MRI. To improve robustness, we will also attempt to consider using specific regions, such as segmented central gland and peripheral prostate zones for classification.

Acknowledgements. This work is supported by the Research Grants Council (RGC) of HK (Ref. No.: 17202317, 17227616, 17206818, 27209515), and Innovation and Technology Commission (Ref. No.: UIM/353).

References

1. Prostate Cancer International Inc. https://prostatecancerinfolink.net/2018/01/09/prostate-cancer-projections-for-2018/. Accessed 02 Apr 2019
2. American Cancer Society Inc. https://www.cancer.org/cancer/prostate-cancer/about/key-statistics.html. Accessed 02 Apr 2019
3. Oberlin, D.T., Casalino, D.D., Miller, F.H., Meeks, J.J.: Dramatic increase in the utilization of multiparametric magnetic resonance imaging for detection and management of prostate cancer. Abdom. Radiol. **42**(4), 1255–1258 (2017)
4. Hassanzadeh, E., Glazer, D.I., Dunne, R.M., Fennessy, F.M., Harisinghani, M.G., Tempany, C.M.: Prostate imaging reporting and data system version 2 (PI-RADS v2): a pictorial review. Abdom. Radiol. **42**(1), 278–289 (2017)
5. Sonn, G.A., Fan, R.E., Ghanouni, P., et al.: Prostate magnetic resonance imaging interpretation varies substantially across radiologists. Eur. Urol. Focus **5**(4), 592–599 (2017)
6. Karimi, D., Ruan, D.: Synergistic combination of learned and hand-crafted features for prostate lesion classification in multiparametric magnetic resonance imaging. In: Descoteaux, M., Maier-Hein, L., Franz, A., Jannin, P., Collins, D.L., Duchesne, S. (eds.) MICCAI 2017. LNCS, vol. 10435, pp. 391–398. Springer, Cham (2017). https://doi.org/10.1007/978-3-319-66179-7_45
7. Liu, S., Zheng, H., Feng, Y., Li, W.: Prostate cancer diagnosis using deep learning with 3D multiparametric MRI. In: Samuel, G.A., Nicholas, A.P. (eds.) Medical Imaging 2017: Computer-Aided Diagnosis. International Society for Optics and Photonics, vol. 10134, p. 1013428 (2017). https://doi.org/10.1117/12.2277121
8. Kiraly, A.P., et al.: Deep convolutional encoder-decoders for prostate cancer detection and classification. In: Descoteaux, M., Maier-Hein, L., Franz, A., Jannin, P., Collins, D.L., Duchesne, S. (eds.) MICCAI 2017. LNCS, vol. 10435, pp. 489–497. Springer, Cham (2017). https://doi.org/10.1007/978-3-319-66179-7_56
9. He, K., Gkioxari, G., Dollár, P., Girshick, R.: Mask r-cnn. In: Proceedings of the IEEE International Conference on Computer Vision, pp. 2961–2969 (2017)
10. Litjens, G., Debats, O., Barentsz, J., Karssemeijer, N., et al.: Computer-aided detection of prostate cancer in MRI. IEEE Trans. Med. Imaging **33**(5), 1083–1092 (2014)

11. Lemaitre, G., Marti, R., Freixenet, J., Vilanova, J.C., Walker, P.M., et al.: Computer-aided detection and diagnosis for prostate cancer based on mono and multi-parametric MRI: a review. Comput. Biol. Med. **60**, 8–31 (2015)
12. Li, C., Xu, C., Gui, C., et al.: Distance regularized level set evolution and its application to image segmentation. IEEE Trans. Image Process. **19**(12), 3243–3254 (2010)
13. Kingma, D.P., Ba, J.: Adam: a method for stochastic optimization. arXiv preprint arXiv: 1412.6980 (2014)
14. Alkadi, R., Taher, F., El-baz, A., Werghi, N.: A Deep Learning-based approach for the detection and localization of prostate cancer in t2 magnetic resonance images. J. Digit. Imaging, 1–15 (2018)

A Novel Deep Learning Framework for Standardizing the Label of OARs in CT

Qiming Yang[1,2], Hongyang Chao[1,2], Dan Nguyen[1],
and Steve Jiang[1(✉)]

[1] Medical Artificial Intelligence and Automation (MAIA) Laboratory,
Department of Radiation Oncology, UT Southwestern Medical Center,
Dallas, TX, USA
steve.jiang@utsouthwestern.edu
[2] School of Data and Computer Science, Sun Yat-sen University,
Guangzhou, GD, China

Abstract. When organs at risk (OARs) are contoured in computed tomography (CT) images for radiotherapy treatment planning, the labels are often inconsistent, which severely hampers the collection and curation of clinical data for research purpose. Currently, data cleaning is mainly done manually, which is time-consuming. The existing methods for automatically relabeling OARs remain unpractical with real patient data, due to the inconsistent delineation and similar small-volume OARs. This paper proposes an improved data augmentation technique according to the characteristics of clinical data. Besides, a novel 3D non-local convolutional neural network is proposed, which includes a decision making network with voting strategy. The resulting model can automatically identify OARs and solve the problems in existing methods, achieving the accurate OAR re-labeling goal. We used partial data from a public head-and-neck dataset (HN_PETCT) for training, and then tested the model on datasets from three different medical institutions. We have obtained the state-of-the-art results for identifying 28 OARs in the head-and-neck region, and also our model is capable of handling multi-center datasets indicating strong generalization ability. Compared to the baseline, the final result of our model achieved a significant improvement in the average true positive rate (TPR) on the three test datasets (+8.27%, +2.39%, +5.53%, respectively). More importantly, the F1 score of small-volume OAR with only 9 training samples increased from 28.63% to 91.17%.

Keywords: Deep learning · Data cleaning · Organ labeling · Voting

1 Introduction

During radiotherapy treatment planning, organs and risk (OARs) are delineated and labeled. Due to the inconsistency of nomenclature even within the same institution, either caused by differences in physician preferences, treatment plans, vendors and different language environments, the existing large amounts of radiotherapy data are unable to be accessed and shared directly. Table 1 demonstrates an example of inconsistency in nomenclature. Although these are 3 patients' data from the same

© Springer Nature Switzerland AG 2019
D. Nguyen et al. (Eds.): AIRT 2019, LNCS 11850, pp. 52–60, 2019.
https://doi.org/10.1007/978-3-030-32486-5_7

dataset, labels for the same structure are very different. Researchers always spend a lot of time on standardizing labels before the data can be analyzed or modeled [16]. To advance the process of standardization of radiation therapy (RT) data, our community has recently proposed standard [7] for radiotherapy data nomenclature. A re-naming tool that automatically standardizes multi-center RT data not only reduces labor and time required for data standardization but also makes it possible to reuse existing large amounts of medical data.

Table 1. Labels in different patients' data.

Patient 1	Patient 2	Patient 3
Parotide D	RT Parotid	PAROTIDE D
GTVggIIID	Mandible	MANDIBULES
Ext 0.5	LT Eye	PLEXUS BR D
nerf opt drt	Cord	NOD
Moelle	LT SUBMANDIBULAR	GL LACR D
Oeil gche	GTV	CERVEAU-
Cerveau	CTV1	NUQUE
External	EXTERNAL	CONF_I PTV3
pt pr	Midline	5412(1DMPO1.1)_1
Tronc cerebral	Brainstem	PEAU
Cristallin G	LT Parotid	CRISTAL G

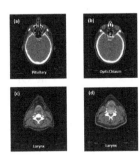

Fig. 1. Delineation in RT. (a) and (b) indicate the similarity of some-volume OARs, (c) and (d) are examples for inconsistent delineation for same OAR.

The related works can be roughly divided into two sets, semi-automatic algorithms and fully automatic algorithms. Mayo et al. [6] developed a software containing structural templates that would help physicians standardizing structures interactively. Recently, Schuler et al. [10] proposed a framework for re-labeling radiotherapy organs by constructing a look-up dictionary that mapping the original labels to standardized labels. The other type of related work, which is based on the invariance of medical image semantics, are learnable automatic recognition method. Rozario et al. [9] used weighted mask of OARs to construct composite mask as 2D input, and trained on a 5-layer convolutional neural network (CNN), which was initial effort towards automated RT data standardization using deep learning (DL).

Simply fixed template or string matching algorithms cannot handle multi-center datasets, there is still a need for manual intervention by physicians. The 5-layer CNN [9] with composite mask as input is not robust enough and does not take into account the problems caused by inconsistent delineation and similar small-volume OARs (see Fig. 1). Hence, these methods still do not meet the application requirements. To improve accuracy and recognition efficiency in multi-center datasets, we proposed a framework based on non-local neural network to automate RT data label standardization, 3DNNV. In the case of limited computational resource, it's capable of overcoming imbalance in training data and efficiently standardizing multi-center RT data with nomenclature recommended in AAPM TG 263 [7].

3D ResNet50 [5] was utilized as the backbone network to enhance the recognition performance of OARs. Compared to other state-of-the-art architectures [1, 11], ResNet [5] requires less computation resource and be capable of achieving higher recognition accuracy on classification task. Then, we added non-local blocks [15] to enhance the representation of global semantic features and ensure the recognition performance of the network. Limited to the size of OARs and computation ability, we proposed a strategy, which performs adaptive sampling and adaptive cropping (ASAC) to generate multi-scale samples, to augment and sampling raw data. In order to make full use of these multi-scale samples and make robust identification, we combined the voting decisions of all scales input of a single sample in inference phase.

In this paper, we highlight our work as followed:

1. An easy and effective data augmentation strategy was applied to improve the accuracy of identifying OARs.
2. We adopt non-local network to construct a novel framework, 3DNNV, with voting strategy to standardize labels in RT data.
3. We tested 3DNNV on multi-center datasets to prove its generalization ability.

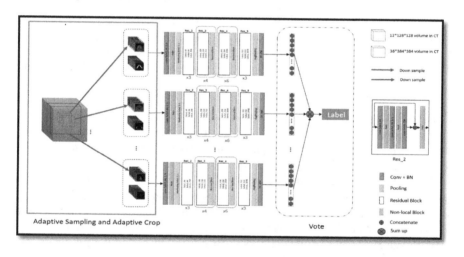

Fig. 2. Architecture of 3DNNV.

2   Materials and Methods

2.1   Dataset

HN_PETCT [12, 13] is an open-source head-and-neck RT dataset released on TCIA [4] with data collected from 4 different French medical institutions containing 298 patient data. In out experiments, 28 categories of organs at risk (OARs) in the head-and-neck area were selected based on [3]. In total, 4372 samples of 28 OARs

(Lens_L/R, Eye_L/R, Glnd_Lacrimal_L/R, Parotid_L/R, Glnd_Submand_L/R, Cavity_Oral, Lips, Bone_Mandible, Cochlea_L/R, Musc_Constrict, Larynx, Esophagus, BrachialPlex_L/R, Thyroid, Brain, Brainstem, Pituitary, OpticChiasm, OpticNrv_L/R and SpinalCord) were collected, and samples were divided into three dataset for training, validation and test in a ratio of 3:1:1. For lacrimal gland and pituitary, only 9 samples are used as training data.

The PDDCA is an open-source RT dataset containing 48 patient data, released by the MICCAI 2015 Segmentation Challenge [8]. This dataset contains only 9 categories of the head-and-neck OARs (Parotid_L/R, Glnd_Submand_L/R, Bone_Mandible, Brainstem, OpticChiasm, and OpticNrv_L/R). All masks are relabelled by trained radiologists. 405 samples of 9 OARs were collected totally, all of which were used as test set.

HN_MAIA is a RT dataset collected by our team and contains data for 406 patients. We collected a total of 5,153 samples of 28 OARs, all of these were used for test.

2.2 Preprocessing

For each given RT data, 3D CT volume and the corresponding masks will be extracted, and then normalize the voxel size in ratio of *vertical voxel size: horizontal voxel size = 0.7680098:1*. We performed trilinear interpolation in resizing. Due to the variety of HU value, we first truncated the HU value to $[-1000, 2500]$ and then normalize it to $[0, 1]$. For the mask, binary $[0, 1]$ matrix was used to represent it directly. In general, mask should be continuous on the vertical axis, but there is a lack of intermediate mask in some training samples, in this case, we will use the nearest mask to fill the missing slice.

2.3 3DNNV

ASAC. In head-and-neck region, the size of OARs are very different (such as 'Brain', 'Pituitary', and 'SpinalCord'), and if the entire CT and mask volumes are directly fed into neural network, will bring a huge cost of computation and storage. ASAC is a way to unify input data under conditions of limited computation resource and imbalanced training dataset. For each pair of pre-processed 3D CT and mask volumes, the same processing steps were adopted, a sliding window was set to slide in the vertical axis, and a cube of size n × m × m were adaptively and intermittently cropped. Five scales for this work, 12 × 128 × 128, 18 × 192 × 192, 24 × 256 × 256, 30 × 320 × 320 and 36 × 384 × 384. Set the sampling interval distance between slices as interval = n /3 × 2, and slide to extract the samples vertically. Resized all of samples into 12 × 128 × 128, which were the final input for 3DNNV. The process of ASAC is shown in Fig. 2.

Non-local Network. Vanilla ResNet50 was used as the backbone network also the baseline model mentioned in Table 2. Next, we added non-local blocks to backbone network to form the final 3D non-local network, as shown in Fig. 2. Inspired by the self-attention mechanism [14], the non-local block was proposed by Xiaolong et al.

[15], able to capture the global dependence in semantic features. It's designed to handle sequential data. In this experiment, the pairwise function f implemented by using the concatenation form. The non-local block in our network is defined as follows:

$$y_i = \frac{1}{C(x)} \sum_{\forall j} f(x_i, x_j) \phi(x_j) \tag{1}$$

$$f(x_i, x_j) = ReLU\left(W_f^\top [\theta(x_i), \mu(x_j)]\right) \tag{2}$$

$$z_i = \sigma(y_i) + x_i \tag{3}$$

Set x and z as the input and output of non-local block, both of them are the same size of $B \times C \times D \times H \times W$. B denotes batch size of input, C represents the number of channel. D, H, W are depth, height and width respectively. Here i is the index of an output position whose response is to be computed, j is the index of all possible positions, and y is intermediate output with the same size as x. All of φ, θ, μ, and σ are $1 \times 1 \times 1$ convolution layers. Operator [.,.] indicates the concatenation operation, W_f is the mapping matrix and converts the concatenated vector to the scalar output. '$+x_i$' indicates identity mapping, the input x_i is added to the transformed y to get the final output z of the non-local block. $C(x)$ is a regularization term, $C(x) = D \times H \times W$.

Voting Strategy. Voting strategy in deep learning is mostly applied in ensemble networks [2], which combines multiple networks to optimize the final decision and needs extra time to train multiple networks. In our proposed framework, we leveraged ASAC to generate multi-scale input data. To make full use of the multi-scale/multi-position information in input data, we combined all the multiscale input of the same sample to vote for a final recognition result in inference phase.

3   Experimental Results

3.1   Setting

Oversampled the minority of OARs to reduce the impact of imbalanced training data and performed affine transformation to augment the training data, includes randomly translate, rotate, shear, and scale, and then cropped the central cube of sample as input data, all of these were implemented on the fly. The final input sample size is $2 \times 12 \times 96 \times 96$, which is two-channel 3D data, includes 3D CT volume and corresponding mask on the same slices. 3DNNV was implemented on the PyTorch 1.0 framework and trained on single GPU NVIDIA Tesla K80. We adopt Adam [17] to optimize the networks with initial learning rate 1e−4. Batch size is set to 16. For the experiments using the samples generated by ASAC, epoch is 20, and the learning rate drops by a factor of 10 after 2, 5, 10 epochs. For other experiments, we set the total number of epoch to 200, and the learning rate decrease by a factor of 10 after 10, 20, 30 epochs. Here, we use cross-entropy loss as the optimization objective function.

3.2   3DNNV vs. Baselines

In the dataset generate by ASAC, the samples collected at the scale of $12 \times 128 \times 128$ are marked as local samples (LS), and the samples collected at the scale of $36 \times 384 \times 384$ are marked as global samples (GS). As shown in Table 2, the normalization of voxel size can reduce the geometric variance of the same category of OAR in different patient data and improve model recognition performance. Baseline (VN-GS) is compared to the baseline (VN-LS), which indicates that local samples are beneficial for identifying small-volume OARs. However, as shown in Fig. 3, the baseline (VN-LS) model exhibits severe confusion in identifying BrachyalPlex_L (BP_L) and BrachyalPlex_R (BP_R), and the confusion is not present in experiments by using global samples. These results indicate that the detailed information in the local sample helps identify small-volume OARs (such as lens, lacrimal glands, etc.), while the information in the global sample helps capture global location relationship and avoids confusing the left and right organs. A non-local network NN (VN-GS) is applied to enhance the representation of high-level semantic features.

In this task, there is a serious deviation in the size of OARs and the number of sample on each category, which requires a trade-off between global location and local detail. Samples that generated by ASAC were used to train the model, while using only global samples to test in NN (ASAC /VN-GS). Figure 4 indicates that model trained with multi-scale samples has improved on identifying some small-volume OARs.

Table 2.   Results of 3DNNV test on three datasets. Baseline (GS) for using global samples (GS), Baseline (VN-GS) and Baseline (VN-LS) are using voxel normalized global samples and local samples.

Architectures	Datesets	TPR	F1-Score	AUC
Baseline (GS)	HN_PETCT	91.54 ± 17.13	91.61 ± 15.96	95.72 ± 8.59
	PDDCA	97.61 ± 5.02	98.51 ± 3.22	98.79 ± 2.55
	HN_MAIA	93.36 ± 9.61	91.81 ± 13.28	96.60 ± 4.82
Baseline (VN-GS)	HN_PETCT	95.33 ± 10.71	95.83 ± 9.00	97.64 ± 5.36
	PDDCA	99.04 ± 2.08	99.43 ± 1.10	99.51 ± 1.03
	HN_MAIA	96.54 ± 5.29	95.75 ± 7.13	98.23 ± 2.65
Baseline (VN-LS)	HN_PETCT	98.56 ± 2.49	98.72 ± 1.93	99.26 ± 1.25
	PDDCA	97.79 ± 6.40	98.69 ± 3.73	98.89 ± 3.20
	HN_MAIA	96.03 ± 6.04	93.96 ± 12.18	97.96 ± 3.07
NN (VN-GS)	HN_PETCT	96.07 ± 7.97	96.27 ± 7.36	98.00 ± 3.99
	PDDCA	98.96 ± 3.12	99.45 ± 1.65	99.48 ± 1.56
	HN_MAIA	96.56 ± 5.15	96.53 ± 4.05	98.24 ± 2.58
NN (ASAC/VN-GS)	HN_PETCT	98.18 ± 4.14	98.59 ± 2.76	99.07 ± 2.06
	PDDCA	99.19 ± 2.29	99.57 ± 1.20	99.59 ± 1.15
	HN_MAIA	98.32 ± 2.26	97.42 ± 5.57	99.13 ± 1.12
3DNNV	HN_PETCT	**99.81 ± 0.63**	**99.82 ± 0.39**	**99.90 ± 0.31**
	PDDCA	**100 ± 0**	**100 ± 0**	**100 ± 0**
	HN_MAIA	**98.87 ± 2.37**	**98.90 ± 1.91**	**99.42 ± 1.19**

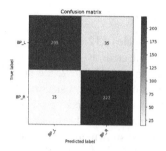

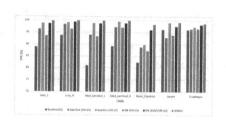

Fig. 3. Confusion matrix

Fig. 4. Some results of OARs in HN_MAIA.

How-
ever, that's still not enough to distinguish Pituitary and OpticChiasm (Shown in Table 3). To further optimize the model and make full use of multi-scale samples, we used voting strategy to optimize the decision-making process to make the recognition results more reliable. Finally, a new framework, 3DNNV, is proposed. Table 3 indicates that the 3DNNV model performed well in identifying small-volume OARs, even they are similar in shape, size and location, after learning scale invariance, global position and local details in the samples.

Table 3. F1-Score (%) of Pituitary and OpticChiasm on HN_MAIA

Methods	Pituitary	OpticChiasm
Baseline (GS)	28.63 ± 8.33	86.35 ± 4.06
Baseline (VN-GS)	61.87 ± 18.73	96.83 ± 1.91
Baseline (VN-LS)	42.61 ± 10.87	90.41 ± 2.38
NN (VN-GS)	82.05 ± 15.77	98.32 ± 0.97
NN (ASAC/VN-GS)	69.67 ± 5.29	97.15 ± 0.67
3DNNV	**91.17 ± 3.18**	**99.47 ± 0.18**

3.3   3DNNV vs. Other Methods

We performed fuzzy string matching algorithm and 5-layer CNN with composite mask to identify the OARs, and compared the performance with 3DNNV. All methods shown in Table 4, were used the same datasets for training and test, except Fuzzy-wuzzy [18], which is not learnable string matching algorithm used all the samples to test. Due to different language environments, only 40.98% on accuracy to map the original labels in HN_PETCT to standardized labels by using string matching method. It turns out that our method are applicable with higher accuracy and generalization ability in multi-center datasets.

Table 4. Average TPR (%) of different methods test on three datasets

Methods	HN_PETCT	PDDCA	HN_MAIA
Fuzzywuzzy [18]	40.98	–	88.74
5-layer CNN [9]	74.28 ± 22.88	58.61 ± 36.58	57.10 ± 25.63
3DNNV	**99.81 ± 0.63**	**100 ± 0**	**98.87 ± 2.37**

4 Conclusions

In this paper, we propose a novel framework, combined with an improved data augmentation method and voting decision-making, which overcoming inconsistent delineation and similar small-volume OARs in imbalanced dataset, to relabel OARs with high accuracy.

References

1. Going deeper with convolutional neural network for intelligent transportation (2016)
2. Battiti, R., Colla, A.M.: Democracy in neural nets: voting schemes for classification. Neural Netw. **7**, 691–707 (1994)
3. Brouwer, C.L., et al.: Ct-based delineation of organs at risk in the head and neck region: Dahanca, eortc, gortec, hknpcsg, ncic ctg, ncri, nrg oncology and trog consensus guidelines. Radiother. Oncol. J. Eur. Soc. Ther. Radiol. Oncol. **117**(1), 83–90 (2015)
4. Clark, K., et al.: The cancer imaging archive (tcia): maintaining and operating a public information repository. J. Digit. Imaging **26**(6), 1045–1057 (2013)
5. He, K., et al.: Deep residual learning for image recognition. In: 2016 IEEE Conference on Computer Vision and Pattern Recognition (CVPR), pp. 770–778 (2016)
6. Mayo, C.S., et al.: Establishment of practice standards in nomenclature and prescription to enable construction of software and databases for knowledge-based practice review. Pract. Radiat. Oncol. **6**(4), e117–e126 (2016)
7. Mayo, C.S., et al.: American association of physicists in medicine task group 263: Standardizing nomenclatures in radiation oncology. Int. J. Radiat. Oncol. Biol. Phys. **100**(4), 1057–1066 (2017)
8. Raudaschl, P., et al.: Evaluation of segmentation methods on head and neck ct: Auto-segmentation challenge 2015. Med. Phys. **44**(5), 2020–2036 (2017)
9. Rozario, T., et al.: Towards automated patient data cleaning using deep learning: A feasibility study on the standardization of organ labeling. CoRR abs/1801.00096 (2017)
10. Schuler, T., et al.: Big data readiness in radiation oncology: an efficient approach for relabeling radiation therapy structures with their tg-263 standard name in realworld data sets. Adv. Radiat. Oncol. **4**(1), 191–200 (2019)
11. Simonyan, K., Zisserman, A.: Very deep convolutional networks for large-scale image recognition. CoRR abs/1409.1556 (2015)
12. Vallières, M., et al.: Radiomics strategies for risk assessment of tumour failure in head-and-neck cancer. Scientific Reports **7**(1), 10117 (2017)
13. Vallières, M., et al.: Data from head-neck-pet-ct. The Cancer Imaging Archive (2017). https://doi.org/10.7937/k9/tcia.2017.8oje5q00
14. Vaswani, A., et al.: Attention is all you need. In: NIPS (2017)

15. Wang, X., et al.: Non-local neural networks. In: 2018 IEEE/CVF Conference on Computer Vision and Pattern Recognition, pp. 7794–7803 (2018)
16. Zhu, W., et al.: Anatomynet: deep learning for fast and fully automated whole volume segmentation of head and neck anatomy. Med. Phy. **46**(2), 576–589 (2018)
17. Kingma, D.P., et al.: Adam: a Method for stochastic optimization. In: ICLR (2015)
18. Jose Diaz-Gonzalez, Fuzzywuzzy (2014). https://github.com/seatgeek/fuzzywuzzy

Multimodal Volume-Aware Detection and Segmentation for Brain Metastases Radiosurgery

Szu-Yeu Hu[1], Wei-Hung Weng[2], Shao-Lun Lu[3], Yueh-Hung Cheng[4],
Furen Xiao[5], Feng-Ming Hsu[3], and Jen-Tang Lu[4(✉)]

[1] Massachusetts General Hospital, Boston, MA, USA
[2] Massachusetts Institute of Technology, Cambridge, MA, USA
[3] Department of Oncology, National Taiwan University Hospital, Taipei, Taiwan
[4] Vysioneer Inc., Cambridge, MA, USA
jt@vysioneer.com
[5] Department of Surgery, National Taiwan University Hospital, Taipei, Taiwan

Abstract. Stereotactic radiosurgery (SRS), which delivers high doses of irradiation in a single or few shots to small targets, has been a standard of care for brain metastases. While very effective, SRS currently requires manually intensive delineation of tumors. In this work, we present a deep learning approach for automated detection and segmentation of brain metastases using multimodal imaging and ensemble neural networks. In order to address small and multiple brain metastases, we further propose a volume-aware Dice loss which optimizes model performance using the information of lesion size. This work surpasses current benchmark levels and demonstrates a reliable AI-assisted system for SRS treatment planning for multiple brain metastases.

Keywords: Brain metastases · Radiosurgery · Deep learning

1 Introduction

Brain metastases (BMs) are the most common intracranial tumors in adults (10 times more common than primary brain tumors) and occur in around 20% of all patients with cancer [5]. The treatment options for brain metastases include craniotomy, chemotherapy, whole brain radiation therapy, and stereotactic radiosurgery (SRS). Among all the options, SRS has been playing a critical role in the treatment of brain metastases as recent studies have shown that SRS leads to better treatment outcomes [10]. By delivering high doses of irradiation in a single or few shots to small targets, SRS effectively destroys tumors without damaging surrounding tissues and has been proved to be beneficial in the local tumor control and post-operative neurocognitive function [3].

S.-Y. Hu and W.-H. Weng—Work done while at Vysioneer.

© Springer Nature Switzerland AG 2019
D. Nguyen et al. (Eds.): AIRT 2019, LNCS 11850, pp. 61–69, 2019.
https://doi.org/10.1007/978-3-030-32486-5_8

As SRS requires precise delineation of tumor margins, target segmentation (contouring) for BMs is performed manually by the radiation oncologist or neuro-surgeon on magnetic resonance images (MRI) and computed tomography (CT) images of the brain. However, such manually contouring process can be very time-consuming and suffer from large inter and intra-reader variability [11]. Driven by the ever-increasing capability of deep learning, automated segmentation of BMs using neural networks has been recently proposed [1,6]. Previous works on computer-aided segmentation of BMs used only MRI as an imaging input. While MRI provides superior ability to characterize neural tissue and the brain structure, MRI is prone to have the problems of spatial distortion and motion artifacts, which can lead to inaccuracy in SRS. CT, on the other hand, is lack of soft tissue contrast but provides a direct measurement of electron densities for radiation dose calculations and has excellent spatial fidelity. Consequently, co-registration between MRI and CT modalities is recommended for precise stereotactic applications [9].

Many previous works on automated segmentation of brain tumors focused on multiforme glioblastoma and glioma, such as BraTS dataset [7], and aims to optimize Dice similarity coefficient (DSC) [8]. Segmentation of brain metastases is more challenging as metastatic lesions can be very small ($< 1000 \ mm^3$) and a large brain metastasis can coexist with multiple small lesions. Conventional DSC is thus not an ideal metric to evaluate brain metastases segmentation because it would be dominant by the large lesion but ignore small metastases. Unfortunately, small BMs are much crucial to SRS since they are more likely to be missed by clinicians.

In this paper, we aim to utilize deep neural networks for automated detection and segmentation of brain metastases. Specifically, we present a deep learning-based system for brain metastases detection and segmentation using multimodal imaging (MRI+CT) and ensemble neural networks, which produces a more reliable result than that would be achieved by a single image modality and/or a single neural network. To address the challenge of small BMs, we further propose a volume-aware Dice loss ($\ell_{\text{vol-dice}}$), which leverages the information of lesion size to optimize overall segmentation.

2   Methods

2.1   Volume-Aware Dice Loss

The Dice loss (ℓ_{dice}), which aims to optimize DSC, has been widely used as a loss function in medical image segmentation task [8] and can be expressed as:

$$\ell_{\text{dice}}(\boldsymbol{g}, \boldsymbol{p}) = -\frac{2\boldsymbol{g}^\top \boldsymbol{p} + \epsilon}{\boldsymbol{p}^\top \boldsymbol{p} + \boldsymbol{g}^\top \boldsymbol{g} + \epsilon}, \tag{1}$$

where $\boldsymbol{p} \in [0,1]^N$ and $\boldsymbol{g} \in \{0,1\}^N$ are the predicted probability vector and the ground truth binary vector for N voxels, respectively. ϵ is a smoothing constant to avoid the denominator being zero.

For binary segmentation problems with similar sizes of lesions, using ℓ_{dice} as the objective function is a fair option as it is normalized by the number of foreground pixels. However, ℓ_{dice} is not an ideal choice when multiple targets are present with the same label but with different sizes, since the loss will be dominant by the larger targets. To address the issue, we proposed a Volume-Aware Dice Loss ($\ell_{\text{vol-dice}}$) that *optimizes the overall segmentation using the information of lesion size*. $\ell_{\text{vol-dice}}$ can be formulated as:

$$\ell_{\text{vol-dice}}\left(\boldsymbol{g}, \boldsymbol{p} \mid W\right) = -\frac{C\boldsymbol{g}^{\top}W\boldsymbol{p} + \epsilon}{\boldsymbol{p}^{\top}\boldsymbol{p} + \boldsymbol{g}^{\top}W\boldsymbol{g} + \epsilon}, \tag{2}$$

where $W \in \mathbb{R}^{N \times N}$ is a diagonal matrix that W_{ii} is a weight related to the volume of the tumor containing the i-th voxel in the ground truth, denoted by $\text{volume}(i)$. $C := 1 + \boldsymbol{g}^{\top}\boldsymbol{g}/\boldsymbol{g}^{\top}W\boldsymbol{g}$ is a normalization constant such that the maximum of $\ell_{\text{vol-dice}}$ is one. In this paper, we consider the form:

$$W_{ii} = \begin{cases} \left(\frac{\lambda}{\text{volume}(i)}\right)^{1/2} & \text{volume}(i) \neq 0, \\ 0 & \text{otherwise} \end{cases},$$

where λ is a reweighting hyper-parameter and can be defined as follows.

1. **Constant Reweight** (CR): λ is a constant (λ_c), such that the weights are simply proportional to the inverse of the square root of tumor volume.
2. **Batch Reweight** (BR): λ is the largest tumor volume in each batch (λ_l); e.g. if the largest tumor in one batch has 1500 voxels, another small tumor with 60 voxels will have a weight of $\sqrt{1500/60} = 5$.

To demonstrate the effects of $\ell_{\text{vol-dice}}$, assume a brain image volume with three ground-truth tumors, each with 1800, 450 and 200 voxels. Using the batch reweight $\ell_{\text{vol-dice}}$, each tumor will have weights 1, 2 and 3, respectively. Suppose the model perfectly predicts the two larger tumors but fails to detect the smallest one. Under such a scenario, ℓ_{dice} is calculated as $-\frac{2 \times (1800 + 450)}{(1800 + 450 + 200) + (1800 + 450)} = -0.957$ and $\ell_{\text{vol-dice}}$ is $-\frac{C \times (1800 + 450 \times 2)}{(1800 + 450 \times 2 + 200 \times 3) + (1800 + 450)} = -0.847$, where $C = 1 + \frac{2450}{3300}$. It illustrates that $\ell_{\text{vol-dice}}$ is more sensitive to the small structures.

2.2 Deep Learning Framework

While the current benchmark for brain metastases segmentation employs MRI imaging only [1,6], CT imaging is an essential reference for clinical treatment planning due to its spatial accuracy. We thus proposed a deep learning framework using multimodal imaging (MRI+CT) and ensemble neural networks for brain metastases detection and segmentation. The framework is shown in Fig. 1. For the ensemble model, we explored two different architectures—3D U-Net and DeepMedic.

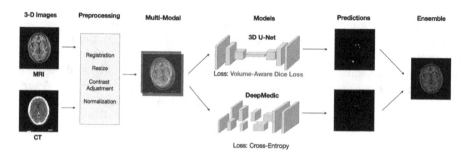

Fig. 1. Proposed deep learning framework with multimodal imaging and ensemble networks.

3D U-Net. 3D U-Net [2] is an extension of the original U-Net by replacing all the 2D operations with 3D counterparts. We added one block in addition to the original implementation (number of feature maps: 32, 64, 128, 256, 512 with convolution kernel size $3 \times 3 \times 3$ and max-pooling size $2 \times 2 \times 1$). We took a full size of the axial-view images and randomly sampled 8 consecutive slices on the vertical axis, resulting in input images size of $512 \times 512 \times 8 \times 2$ (height × width × number of slices × number of imaging modality). We set a limit to ensure that in each epoch, at least 70% of the samples should contain tumor labels. All the 3D U-Net models were trained using a rmsprop optimizer, with learning rate 10^{-3}, batch size of 1, over 300 epochs on an NVIDIA V100 GPU. The best weights on the validation set was used to evaluate the final results on the test set.

DeepMedic. DeepMedic [4] is originally designed for brain tumor segmentation on multi-channel MRI and also had been applied to BMs [1,6]. It consists of multiple parallel pathways—one branch takes small patches from full resolution images as input and the others utilizes subsampled-version of the images. Different from the original paper, the DeepMedic architecture we used contained 3 parallel convolutional pathways, one of which was with normal image resolution and the other two of which were with low resolution using down-sampling factors of 3 and 5. There were 11 layers in the network, the first 8 of which were convolutional layers (number of feature maps: 30, 30, 40, 40, 40, 40, 50, 50 with $3 \times 3 \times 3$ kernels) and the last 3 of which were fully connected layers (with 250 feature maps per layer). The network was trained using a rmsprop optimizer, with learning rate 10^{-3}, minimizing the cross-entropy loss over 35 epochs.

Ensemble Model. 3D U-Net and DeepMedic were trained separately with different hyperparameters and different objective functions to maximize the capability of the ensemble model. While U-Net utilized the full field of view for each image slice and addressed overall tumor segmentation, DeepMedic leveraged image segments during model training and focused on small metastases. Furthermore, U-Net was trained to optimize DSC and DeepMedic was set to minimize cross-entropy loss. At testing time, each model individually generated probability maps of brain metastases. An ensemble confidence map was then created by calculating the average of the predictions of both models.

3 Experiments and Results

Data

The primary cohort for model training and testing consists of 305 patients with 864 brain metastases (median volume 760 mm^3, range 3–110,000 mm^3) treated by CyberKnife G4 system in a single medical center. Each case contains volume masks of brain tumors delineated by an attending radiation oncologist or neurosurgeon on associated CT and T1-weighted MRI scan with contrast. The dataset was split into training (80%), validation (10%), and test set (10%) randomly. To evaluate the model robustness and generalizability, we collected an additional batch of test set from the same institution, containing 36 patients with 96 metastases (median volume 829 mm^3). The results presented in this paper are the average of the two test sets.

For each case, after rigid image registration between CT and MRI image volumes, each slice was resized into 512×512 pixels with the resolution of 0.6 mm $\times$ 0.6 mm, while slice thickness was resampled to 2 mm. Brain window and adaptive histogram equalization were applied to the CT and MRI images slice-by-slice, respectively. All the image volumes were then standardized with zero-mean and unit-variance normalization.

3.1 Volume-Aware Dice Loss

$\ell_{\text{vol-dice}}$ **with Different Reweight Strategies.** We evaluated the efficacy of $\ell_{\text{vol-dice}}$ on the 3D U-Net. A standard 3D U-Net using the multimodal learning (MRI+CT) and conventional ℓ_{dice} was trained as the baseline model. Then we compared the relative change of DSC, precision and recall using different settings of $\ell_{\text{vol-dice}}$. In the combination of two test sets, the tumors has median 1322 voxels (949 mm^3) and mean 4721 voxels (3389 mm^3). We tested the λ_c of 500, 1000, 2500, 5000 for the CR strategy.

Our baseline model achieves a DSC of 0.669, precision 0.689 and recall 0.700. Table 1 lists the results of applying $\ell_{\text{vol-dice}}$ relative to the baseline. Overall, using the $\ell_{\text{vol-dice}}$ with BR (λ_l) yields the best performance, improving 8.57% of DSC and 24.14% of recall compared to the baseline. The performance of $\ell_{\text{vol-dice}}$ with CR largely depends on the constant value; the higher the constant, the better the recalls. Such an observation is consistent with our expectation that the $\ell_{\text{vol-dice}}$ focuses more on easily neglected small structures and has a higher sensitivity. However, in our dataset, the tumor sizes are highly diverse, therefore making it challenging to determine a value that can generalize to all the tumors. On the other hand, the BR approach has more flexibility using a dynamic weighting strategy, which provides a balance between precision and recall.

Table 1. Performance of different configurations with $\ell_{vol\text{-}dice}$. All the models were trained on 3D U-Net with CT and MRI.

$\ell_{vol\text{-}dice}$ configuration		Metric Change over ℓ_{dice} loss (%)		
Reweight method	λ	DSC	Precision	Recall
Batch-reweight	-	**+8.57%**	+2.62%	+24.14%
Const-reweight	$\lambda_c = 500$	−52.11%	+2.78%	−70.08%
Const-reweight	$\lambda_c = 1000$	−7.67%	**+13.15%**	−18.83%
Const-reweight	$\lambda_c = 2500$	+2.22%	−5.55%	+23.04%
Const-reweight	$\lambda_c = 5000$	−8.60%	−31.68%	**+25.46%**

Table 2. Pixel-wise and metastasis-wise recall

Tumor	Numbers	Median size	Loss	Pixel-wise recall	Metastasis-wise recall
Small ($\leq 1500\,\mathrm{mm}^3$)	113	368	ℓ_{dice}	0.466	0.619
			$\ell_{vol\text{-}dice}$	0.633	0.672
Large ($>1500\,\mathrm{mm}^3$)	78	4114	ℓ_{dice}	0.826	0.987
			$\ell_{vol\text{-}dice}$	0.828	0.974

$\ell_{vol\text{-}dice}$ **on Small Tumors.** To evaluate the effectiveness of $\ell_{vol\text{-}dice}$ on different sizes of lesions, we further divided the lesions into large and small tumor groups at a cut-off point of 1500 mm^3. We calculated (1) pixel-wise recall, and (2) tumor-wise recall, where a positive tumor prediction is defined as detected if there is at least one pixel being predicted; noted that we did not measure the DSC and the precision because the false positive pixels can't be categorized into either small or large tumors easily. The results are shown in Table 2. $\ell_{vol\text{-}dice}$ shows a more significant improvement in the small tumor groups, increasing the recall from 0.466 to 0.633 and detection rate from 0.619 to 0.672; while in the large tumor groups, the performances of the two settings are almost identical. The results indicate that the $\ell_{vol\text{-}dice}$ effectively improve the recall in the small tumors.

3.2   Deep Learning Framework

In our final proposed deep learning framework, we used (1) multimodal learning adopting MRI+CT, (2) ensemble learning considering 3D U-Net and DeepMedic, and (3) optimization using $\ell_{vol\text{-}dice}$.

As shown in Table 3, 3D U-Net and DeepMedic obtain a DSC of 0.669 and 0.625 respectively. DeepMedic utilizes a patch-based training method, which makes the network focusing on smaller regions and contributing to a higher recall; on the other hand, 3D U-Net takes full resolution as inputs. The advantage of seeing the complete brain structure leads to higher precision. The ensemble

Table 3. Model performance of different configurations of loss functions, image modalities, and neural network models. The values are represented as median (std).

Model	$\ell_{\text{vol-dice}}$	DSC	Precision	Recall
3D U-Net		0.669 (0.006)	0.689 (0.001)	0.700 (0.015)
DeepMedic		0.625 (0.013)	0.631 (0.004)	0.734 (0.035)
3D U-Net + DeepMedic		0.719 (0.004)	**0.788** (0.002)	0.713 (0.023)
3D U-Net + DeepMedic	✓	**0.740** (0.022)	0.779 (0.010)	**0.803** (0.001)

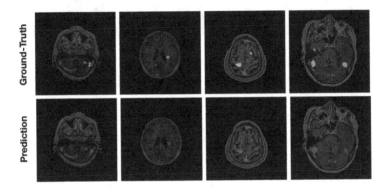

Fig. 2. Examples of the prediction results overlaying with MRI.

of the two models improves the DSC to 0.719. Further applying the $\ell_{\text{vol-dice}}$ (with BR) on 3D U-Net, we achieve the best DSC of 0.740 and recall of 0.803. The results indicate that our deep learning approach effectively increases the DSC, precision, and recall. The performance surpasses the current benchmark methods. Examples of prediction results are shown in Fig. 2.

3.3 Limitation

As the annotations were carried out by the neurosurgeon or radiation oncologist during SRS treatment planning, the ground truth labels represent the area for the treatment rather than the actual tumor extent, which leads to imperfect annotations for tumor segmentation. Based on the clinician's experience and the patient's disease status, these annotations can be delineated more aggressively or conservatively. Figure 3(a) illustrates an example of an aggressive treatment planning, which shows a broader area than the lesion. Also, the clinician would ignore previously treated tumors (Fig. 3(b)). Last, some difficult cases, such as Fig. 3(c) and (d), are highly subjective and should be determined through clinical manifestations or the series change of MRI. The cases mentioned above can underestimate our model performance and lead to a higher variance.

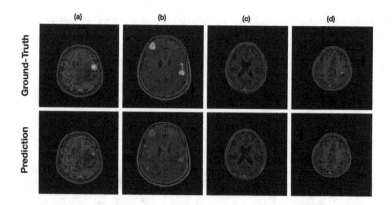

Fig. 3. Examples of failed cases overlaying with MRI.

4   Conclusion

In this paper, we have achieved high performance for automated detection and segmentation of brain metastases, utilizing multimodal imaging (MRI+CT) as inputs and ensemble neural networks. We have also addressed the challenge of lesion size variance in multiple metastases by introducing a volume-aware Dice loss, which leverages the information of lesion size and significantly enhances the overall segmentation and sensitivity of small lesions, which are critical in the current SRS contouring workflow. It is expected that the proposed solution will facilitate tumor contouring and treatment planning of stereotactic radiosurgery.

References

1. Charron, O., Lallement, A., Jarnet, D., Noblet, V., Clavier, J.B., Meyer, P.: Automatic detection and segmentation of brain metastases on multimodal mr images with a deep convolutional neural network. Comput. Biol. Med. **95**, 43–54 (2018)
2. Çiçek, Ö., Abdulkadir, A., Lienkamp, S.S., Brox, T., Ronneberger, O.: 3D U-Net: learning dense volumetric segmentation from sparse annotation. In: Ourselin, S., Joskowicz, L., Sabuncu, M.R., Unal, G., Wells, W. (eds.) MICCAI 2016. LNCS, vol. 9901, pp. 424–432. Springer, Cham (2016). https://doi.org/10.1007/978-3-319-46723-8_49
3. Hartgerink, D.E., et al.: Stereotactic radiosurgery in the management of patients with brain metastases of non-small cell lung cancer; indications, decision tools and future directions. Front. Oncol. **8**, 154 (2018)
4. Kamnitsas, K., et al.: Efficient multi-scale 3D CNN with fully connected crf for accurate brain lesion segmentation. Med. Image Anal. **36**, 61–78 (2017)
5. Lin, X., DeAngelis, L.M.: Treatment of brain metastases. J. Clin. Oncol. **33**(30), 3475 (2015)
6. Liu, Y., et al.: A deep convolutional neural network-based automatic delineation strategy for multiple brain metastases stereotactic radiosurgery. PloS One **12**(10), e0185844 (2017)

7. Menze, B.H., et al.: The multimodal brain tumor image segmentation benchmark (brats). IEEE Trans. Med. Imaging **34**(10), 1993–2024 (2015)
8. Milletari, F., Navab, N., Ahmadi, S.A.: V-net: fully convolutional neural networks for volumetric medical image segmentation. In: 2016 Fourth International Conference on 3D Vision (3DV), pp. 565–571. IEEE (2016)
9. Pereira, G.C., Traughber, M., Muzic, R.F.: The role of imaging in radiation therapy planning: past, present, and future. BioMed Res. Int. **2014** (2014)
10. Tsao, M.N., et al.: Radiotherapeutic and surgical management for newly diagnosed brain metastasis (es): an American society for radiation oncology evidence-based guideline. Pract. Radiat. Oncol. **2**(3), 210–225 (2012)
11. Vinod, S.K., Jameson, M.G., Min, M., Holloway, L.C.: Uncertainties in volume delineation in radiation oncology: a systematic review and recommendations for future studies. Radiother. Oncol. **121**(2), 169–179 (2016)

Voxel-Level Radiotherapy Dose Prediction Using Densely Connected Network with Dilated Convolutions

Jingjing Zhang[1], Shuolin Liu[1], Teng Li[1(✉)], Ronghu Mao[2], Chi Du[3], and Jianfei Liu[1]

[1] Electrical Engineering and Automation, Anhui University, Hefei, China
tenglwy@gmail.com
[2] Radiation Oncology, The Affiliated Cancer Hospital of Zhengzhou University, Zhengzhou, China
[3] Cancer Center, The Second Peoples Hospital of Neijiang, Sichuan, China

Abstract. Radiotherapy treatment planning often demands substantial manual adjustments to achieve maximal dose delivery at the planning target volumes (PTVs) and protecting surrounding organs at risk (OARs). Automatic dose prediction can reduce manual adjustments by providing close to optimal radiotherapy planning parameters, which is studied in this work. We developed a voxel-level dose prediction framework based on an end-to-end trainable densely-connected network. We designed a four-channel map to record the geometric features of PTVs, OARs, and the prescription dose of each patient. The densely connected block was modified with dilated convolutions to catch multi-scale features, which can result in accurate dense prediction. 90 esophageal radiation treatment plans from 90 patients were used in this work (72 plans used for training and the remaining 18 plans for testing). Average value of mean absolute error of dose volume histogram (DVH) and voxel-based mean absolute error were used to evaluate the prediction accuracy, with [0.9%, 1.9%] at PGTV, [1.1%, 2.8%] at PTV, [2.8%, 4.4%] at Lung, [3.5%, 6.9%] at Heart, [4.2%, 5.6%] at Spinal Cord, and [1.7%, 4.8%] at Body. These encouraging results demonstrated that the proposed framework could provide accurate dose prediction, which could be very useful to guide radiotherapy treatment planning.

Keywords: Radiation therapy · Dose prediction · Convolutional neural networks · Dilated convolution · Densely-connected network

This work is supported by the National Natural Science Foundation of China (No. 61702001), and the Anhui Provincial Natural Science Foundation of China (No. 1908085J25) (No. 1808085MF209), and Key Support Program of University Outstanding Youth Talent of Anhui Province (No. gxyqZD2018007), and Open fund for Discipline Construction, Institute of Physical Science and Information Technology, Anhui University.

D. Nguyen et al. (Eds.): AIRT 2019, LNCS 11850, pp. 70–77, 2019.
https://doi.org/10.1007/978-3-030-32486-5_9

1   Introduction

Radiotherapy is one of the major cancer treatment approaches. Radiotherapy treatment planning is a process of adjusting optimization planning parameters, which are highly dependent on the physicists experience. It could potentially demand extensive adjustment and time consumption. One solution is to predict these optimization parameters by extracting knowledge of radiotherapy dose maps (as shown in Fig. 1) from existing plans. The predicted parameters could be a useful reference for physicists to reduce planning time.

The last decade has seen substantial progress in radiotherapy dose prediction. The majority of these work is focusing on the prediction of dose volume histogram (DVH). Principal component analysis and support vector regression were utilized to predict DVH of prostate and head-and-neck radiotherapy based on the observation that DVH is highly correlated with distance between PTVs and OARs [1]. In DVH prediction, spatial features of organs-at-risk (OARs), shape of planning target volumes (PTV), distance-to-target histograms (DTH), overlapping volume histograms (OVHs), etc, are extracted to analyze the relationships between optimal plans. The major limitation of DVH prediction is lacking the prediction of three-dimensional dose distributions. To address this problem, artificial neural network was employed to predict voxel-level dose distribution for pancreatic and prostate patients, which learned more complex relationships between the handcrafted features mentioned above [2]. However, it is remained to be discussed which features infect dose distribution most, and whether other features infect dose distributions are ignored. Recently, convolutional neural network (CNN) based approaches show superior performance in prediction accuracy and training complexity. U-like convolutional neural network was utilized to predict dose distribution of head and neck cancer patients, where labeled PTVs and OARs were sent to the network and three-dimensional dose prediction was generated [3]. In U-like convolutional neural network, a stack of down-sampling operations were used to reduce the resolution of feature maps and achieve larger receptive field, which poses serious challenges to preserve the details of small objects such as spinal cord.

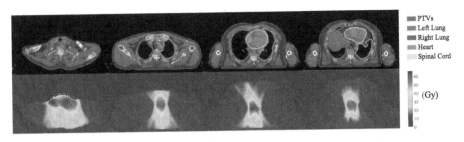

Fig. 1. Examples of some planning regions and their corresponding dose distributions. *Top*: Planning regions, where the anatomy of planning target volumes (PTVs) and organ-at-risks (OARs) are annotated. *Bottom*: Dose maps where the value of each pixel records the dose value of a certain voxel by the unit of Gary (Gy).

In this paper, we provide a novel approach for voxel-level dose prediction. Specifically, a four-channel map was develop as the input to the system, where the information of PTVs, OARs, and the prescription from doctors are recorded. Then, we used a improved U-like architecture with a adapted dense block [4]. To effectively enlarge the receptive field, which could catch more details and result in accurate dense prediction. Our contributions could be summarized as follows: (1) We introduce a novel four-channel input to dose prediction task, which could preserve the factors which may infect dose distribution in the maximum degree. (2) We specially design a convolutional neural network for dose prediction task. We drop most of the down-sampling operations and employ an improved dense block with dilated convolutions to catch multi-scale features and achieve accurate dense prediction. (3) The entire network is end-to-end trainable. Dose maps (such as Fig. 1) could be generated slice by slice without any manual intervention, where the value of each pixel records the dose value of a certain voxel.

2   Method

2.1   Input to the System

The prescription dose of each target volume, spatial information of PTVs and OARs are transformed to a four-channel map (analogous to how RGB images are treated as three separate channels).

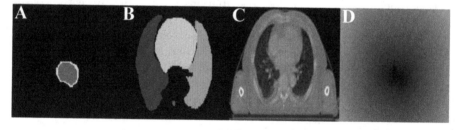

Fig. 2. (A) Planning gross target volume (PGTV) and planning target volume (PTV) fixed with their corresponding prescription dose. (B) Organs-at-risk signed with unique labels, form 1 to 4. (C) CT scans. (D) D-img where the value of each pixel records its' distance to PTV boundary.

In order to describe the prescriptions from doctors and the spatial information of PTVs, we fixed the areas of PTVs with their prescription dose (see Fig. 2A), which could be described as $P_1 A + P_2(A - B)$, where A, B are the binary mask of planning gross target volume (PGTV) and planning target volume (PTV), and P_1, P_2 are their corresponding prescription dose. In Fig. 2B, the organ-at-risks is distinguished by labeling various numbers (from 1 to 4). These labels of organs are used to help recognize the geometric features such as their location, shape, size, spatial association to target volume, etc, which are supplementary to conventional features from CT scans. The CT scans were also sent to the networks to provide more details (see Fig. 2C). Since dose distributions outside beam field drops fastly, we use a distance image(named D-img for short) to supplement details for distinguishing the locations of each voxel. In D-img, the value of each pixel records the distance from each voxel to the boundary of PTV(as shown in Fig. 2D). Considering the in-plane resolution of CT scans varies between 0.90 mm and 1.37 mm per pixel, adding D-img to input could also help retain this information. Generally, the value of pixel (x,y,z) in D-img is :

$$f(x, y, z) = \min_{C_i \subset \Omega_c} \|(x, y, z), C_j\| \tag{1}$$

while Ω_c is the contour set of the planned target volumes (PTVs).

2.2   Model Architecture

Our model architecture is adapted based on U-Net, which is shown in Fig. 3. It employed classic encode-decode architecture. The encoding stage used some similar blocks, which consist of two 3×3 convolutions, a rectified linear unit (ReLU) and a 2×2 max pooling operation. Different from standard U-Net, we only employed two max pooling operations to reduced the resolution of feature maps, which means the size of feature maps are at least 64×64. We double the number of feature channels after down-sampling operation. After a dense block, The decoding stage gradually up-sampling the feature maps to the original resolution by 2×2 deconvolutions with stride of 2. At the final layer a 1×1 convolution is used to reduce the channels of features to 1 and generate predicted dose map. In practice, We chose 32 as the basic number of channels, which is suitable for our data size (90 cases).

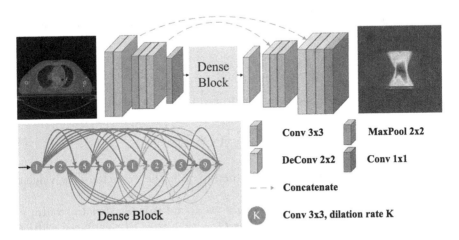

Fig. 3. Schematic of an example architecture used for dose prediction, which consist of convolution layers, deconvolution layers, max pooling layers, and a dense block. The numbers in dense block represent the dilation rate of each convolution operation. The input to the network is a four-channel map we introduced in Sect. 2.1, while the output of the network is the dose map.

Multi-scale Features Aggregation. In order to effectively enlarge the receptive field and catch multi-scale features, we employed dilated convolutions, a powerful tool in dense prediction tasks, as the basic unit of dense block. We followed the idea of Yang et al. to avoid gridding issue [5]. When we designed the block with hybrid dilated convolutions. The dilation rates of 3×3 convolutions are repeated by a sequence of 1, 2, 5, and 9, their corresponding receptive field could varies to 3×3, 5×5, 11×11, 19×19. This mechanism allows us to effectively enlarge the receptive field without down-sampling operations. Besides, dilated convolutions have the same number of parameters as the original 3×3 convolutions. Let denote the 3×3 convolution kernel that related to layer $\mathcal{L}^{\ell}$ by $\mathcal{K}^{\ell}$, then dilated convolutions could describes as follow:

$$(\mathcal{L}^{\ell} *_d \mathcal{K}^{\ell})(\boldsymbol{p}) = \sum_{a+db=p} \mathcal{L}^{\ell}(a)\mathcal{K}^{\ell}(b) \tag{2}$$

where $\boldsymbol{p}$ is the domain of feature maps in $\mathcal{L}^{\ell}$, $*_d$ is the discrete convolution operator with dilation rate of d.

Design of Dense Block. To ensure maximum information flow, all layers are directly connected with their frontal layers in our dense block. Our dense block composed of 8 dilated convolution layers. Generally, let denote the output of ℓth layer in dense block by $\mathcal{X}^{\ell}$, specially $\mathcal{X}^0$ is the input of dense block, and denote $\mathcal{H}(.)$ as a non-linear transformation, which composed of convolution operations and point-wise truncations max(., 0). Then the output of each layer in dense block could be represented as:

$$\mathcal{X}^{\ell} = \mathcal{H}([X^0, X^1, \ldots, X^{\ell-1}]), \ \ell = 1, 2, \ldots, 8. \tag{3}$$

Thanks to the dense connections, the whole network is easy to train and have highly efficient parameters [4].

2.3   Optimization

Mean square error calculated according to Eq. 4 is employed as the loss function.

$$L = \frac{1}{N}\sum_i^N \frac{1}{2}(y_i - \hat{y}_i)^2 \tag{4}$$

where N is the total voxel of target structure, y_i is the predicted dose value of ith voxel, $\hat{y}_i$ is the clinical dose value.

Training was conducted in two stages, we found it is beneficial to warm up the framework with some similar slices $Q = \{z \mid z_k - 10 \leq z \leq z_k + 10\}$ of each patient for the first 1000 iterations, where z_k is the approximate sequence number of the slice which located on the middle of chest. Then, we trained the network with all the slices for 100 epochs. Standard stochastic gradient descent (SGD) with batch size 1, momentum $\beta = 0.99$ and weight decay $\omega = 0.0005$ was used for optimization. All the experiments were running with Caffe library.

2.4 Data Collection and Validation Methods

A total of 90 plans of esophagus cancer patients treated with single arc volumetric modulated arc therapy at 6 MV were collected in our research, all treatment plans are optimized and clinical accepted. The size of planning target volumes varying between 88.3 cm³ and 1051.4 cm³, the median size is 516.9 cm³. The in-plane resolution of CT scans varying between 0.90 mm and 1.37 mm per pixel, and slice thickness is 5 mm.

In order to evaluate the general level of prediction accuracy, we employed mean absolute error of dose volume histogram (MAE$_D$) calculated according to Eq. 5, voxel-based mean absolute error (MAE$_V$) calculated according to Eq. 6, as the evaluation materials.

$$MAE_D = \frac{1}{99} \sum_{i=1}^{99} |d(i) - \hat{d}(i)| / prescription\ dose \times 100\% \tag{5}$$

$$MAE_V = \frac{1}{n} \sum_{j=1}^{n} |v(j) - \hat{v}(j)| / prescription\ dose \times 100\% \tag{6}$$

D_n is denoted as the dose that n% of the volume of a region of interest is at least receiving, $d(i)$ is the predicted D_i while $\hat{d}(i)$ is the true D_i, n is the number of total voxel, $v(j)$ is the predicted dose value of jth voxel while $\hat{v}(j)$ is the true dose of jth voxel.

We employed 5-fold cross-validation procedure (72 cases for training and 18 cases for testing) in the evaluation stage and calculate the mean value as the final score.

3 Experimental Results

Considering patients' data and treatment modalities are diverse, we reproduce U-net dose prediction approach on our dataset for comparison. Besides, we also evaluate the performance of the situations with or without D-img to stress its' importance.

Table 1. The average scores of MAE$_D$ of different structures (include PGTV, PTV, lung, heart, spinal cord).

Method	MAE$_D$ (PGTV)(%)	MAE$_D$ (PTV)(%)	MAE$_D$ (Lung)(%)	MAE$_D$ (Heart)(%)	MAE$_D$ (Cord)(%)	MAE$_D$ (Body)(%)
U-net	0.9±0.9	1.2±0.6	3.5±2.8	4.4±4.1	6.2±3.9	2.3±1.8
Ours	1.1±1.3	1.4±1.2	2.8±3.6	3.7±4.5	5.5±7.5	1.8±1.6
Ours+D-img	**0.9±0.8**	**1.1±0.7**	**2.8±2.7**	**3.5±4.5**	**4.2±6.5**	**1.7±1.3**

Overall, as showed in Tables 1 and 2, our predictions show high accuracy. As a typical prediction example, Fig. 4 shows an intuitive comparison of DVH

Table 2. The average scores of MAE$_V$ of different structures (include PGTV, PTV, lung, heart, spinal cord).

Method	MAE$_V$ (PGTV)(%)	MAE$_V$ (PTV)(%)	MAE$_V$ (Lung)(%)	MAE$_V$ (Heart)(%)	MAE$_V$ (Cord)(%)	MAE$_V$ (Body)(%)
U-net	2.0±0.6	3.0±0.5	5.6±2.8	8.7±6.0	8.3±4.3	5.8±2.5
Ours	2.2±0.8	3.1±0.5	4.9±4.3	8.3±3.8	7.5±3.2	5.5±2.4
Ours+D-img	**1.9±0.3**	**2.8±0.7**	**4.4±3.6**	**6.9±5.1**	**5.6±5.6**	**4.8±2.7**

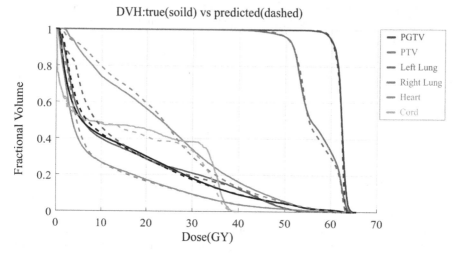

Fig. 4. Example of a typical dose volume histogram (DVH) comparing true dose and predicted dose for one patient, solid lines are the dose volume histogram calculated form clinical dose distribution while dashed line are calculated from our prediction.

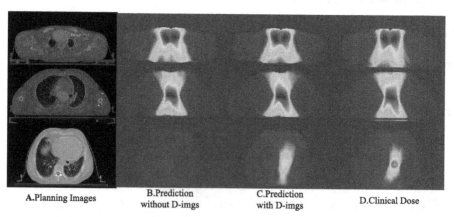

A.Planning Images | B.Prediction without D-imgs | C.Prediction with D-imgs | D.Clinical Dose

Fig. 5. Examples of dose predictions of several slices with vastly different location. (A) The planning regions. (B) The prediction of our framework without combination. (C) The Prediction of our framework with D-img. (D) Their corresponding clinical dose distributions.

between prediction and the true one. Although the prediction error of the spinal cord expresses a slight increase when compared to other structures, the predicted error of the max dose value of spinal cord ($Cord_{max}$), the main quality index to evaluate the dose distributions of spinal cord, is small (1.2%). It means our designing of model architecture and transforming of clinical information are efficient and still clinical acceptable.

Visually on Fig. 5, for those slices which do not contain PTVs but still have complex dose distribution, the model without D-img shows limited ability. The predictions of these edge slices are inaccurate, while adding D-img as input can notably alleviate this issue. According to Tables 1 and 2, the employment of D-img also makes our predictions much more accurate.

4   Conclusion and Future Work

In this study, we proposed a new approach for dose distribution task, which could provide voxel-level dose predictions. The proposed model shows significant improving in prediction accuracy of OARs while achieves comparable or better performance in prediction accuracy of PTVs. The design of the input to the system, especially the design of D-img, was proved to be beneficial for more accurate dose prediction. Overall, using proposed approaches, we are able to accurately predict the dose distribution of all structures within 7% average mean error. These encouraging results demonstrated that the proposed framework could provide accurate dose prediction, which could be very useful to guide radiotherapy treatment planning. In the future, we plan to extend our research by building a beam-filed-attentioned network for automatic treatments planning. Besides, automatic segmentation of organs-at-risks (OARs), detection of plan-target volumes (PTVs), and dose prediction may integrated together in one framework. We expect this research will further provide convenience for clinical planning and research.

References

1. Yuan, L., Ge, Y., Lee, W.R., Yin, F.F., Kirkpatrick, J.P., Wu, Q.J.: Quantitative analysis of the factors which affect the interpatient organ-at-risk dose sparing variation in IMRT plans. Med. Phys. **39**(11), 6868–6878 (2012)
2. Shiraishi, S., Moore, K.L.: Knowledge-based prediction of three-dimensional dose distributions for external beam radiotherapy. Med. Phys. **43**(1), 378–387 (2016)
3. Nguyen, D., et al.: 3D radiotherapy dose prediction on head and neck cancer patients with a hierarchically densely connected U-net deep learning architecture. Phys. Med. Biol. **64**(6), 065020 (2019)
4. Huang, G., Liu, Z., Van Der Maaten, L., Weinberger, K.Q.: Densely connected convolutional networks. In: Proceedings of the IEEE Conference on Computer Vision and Pattern Recognition (CVPR), pp. 2261–2269 (2017)
5. Wang, P., et al.: Understanding convolution for semantic segmentation. In: IEEE Winter Conference on Applications of Computer Vision (WACV), pp. 1451–1460 (2018)

Online Target Volume Estimation and Prediction from an Interlaced Slice Acquisition - A Manifold Embedding and Learning Approach

John Ginn[✉], James Lamb, and Dan Ruan

University of California Los Angeles, Los Angeles, CA 90095, USA
jginn@mednet.ucla.edu

Abstract. In radiotherapy it is critical to have access to real-time volumetric information to support online dose calculation and motion management. MRI-guidance offers an online imaging platform but is restricted by image acquisition speed. This work alleviates this limitation by integrating processing techniques with an interlaced 2D real-time acquisition protocol. We characterize the volumetric anatomical states as samples on a manifold, and consider the alternating 2D slice acquisition as observation models. We infer sample locations in the manifold from partial observations and extrapolate on the manifold to generate real-time target predictions. A series of 10 adjacent images were repeatedly acquired at three frames per second in an interleaved fashion using a 0.35 T MRI-guided radiotherapy system. Eight volunteer studies were performed during free breathing utilizing normal anatomical features as targets. Locally linear embedding (LLE) was combined with manifold alignment to establish correspondence across slice positions. Multislice target contours were generated using a LLE-based motion model for each real-time image. Motion predictions were performed using a weighted k-nearest neighbor based inference with respect to the underlying volume manifold. In the absence of a 3D ground-truth, we evaluate the part of the volume where the acquisition is available retrospectively. The dice similarity coefficient and centroid distance were on average 0.84 and 1.75 mm respectively. This work reports a novel approach and demonstrates promise to achieve volumetric quantifications from partial image information online.

Keywords: Dimensionality reduction · Motion modeling · Motion prediction

1 Introduction

Motion is a critical consideration in radiotherapy. Online MR imaging provides the opportunity to monitor tumor motion during treatment, but imaging techniques are not currently able to acquire volumetric images fast enough to monitor

© Springer Nature Switzerland AG 2019
D. Nguyen et al. (Eds.): AIRT 2019, LNCS 11850, pp. 78–85, 2019.
https://doi.org/10.1007/978-3-030-32486-5_10

the motion of the entire tumor in real-time. Only a portion of the target is visible at each time point and there is no standardized or justified optimization method to select the physical location or cross section of the target that should be monitored during treatment. In addition to obtaining volumetric characterization, it is particularly important to perform prediction to compensate for computational and mechanical latencies to make adaptive adjustment.

Endeavors have been made to use motion models to obtain 3D motion in real-time. Proposed methods include use of a motion lookup table, fitting prior 4D MRI motion to match newly acquired 2D images, manifold learning and use of a bilinear motion model with a respiratory surrogate [1–3,7]. Other relevant works have restricted prediction to 2D setups using autoregressive linear models, support vector machines and kalman filters [7,9]. To our knowledge, only one existing work addressed both limitations simultaneously, predicting motion across multiple slice positions using a respiratory surrogate and lookup table [7].

In this study we propose a unified framework to provide volumetric motion information and perform motion prediction. We utilize a locally linear embedding and manifold alignment technique to simultaneously model motion across multiple imaging planes [2]. We extract and estimate the underlying nonlinear manifold structure of anatomical motion across multiple slice positions and infer the volumetric target descriptor using the manifold for each acquired 2D image to obtain its 3D counterpart and perform real-time volumetric prediction.

2   Methods and Materials

2.1   State Embedding and Manifold Alignment from 2D Images at Different Acquisition Locations

Let $\mathbf{X}$ indicate samples in the ambient space (*i.e.*, 2D images, possibly from different locations), $\mathbf{Y}$ the low-dimensional embedding, W the weights. Further, we will use subscript l to index slice location, so that $\mathcal{X}_l$ $\mathcal{Y}_l$ indicate the collection of ambient samples collected at location l and their corresponding embedding. We utilize an estimation scheme to obtain $\mathcal{Y}_l, l = 1, 2, \ldots, L$ by performing manifold alignment during local linear embedding [1].

As a preprocessing step, for any specific image location l, and each sample i, the K most similar images under the same acquisition condition l are identified and their weights estimated by minimizing

$$\underset{W}{arg\,min} \sum_{i=1}^{N} \left| \mathbf{X}_i - \sum_{j \in \Omega(i)} W_{ij} \mathbf{X}_j \right|^2 . \tag{1}$$

Where $\Omega(i)$ is the index set for the neighborhood, and W_{ij} are the reconstruction weights associated with each nearest neighbor.

Subsequently, we consider a process to generate the embedding by considering both point-wise embedding accuracy and manifold alignment simultaneously. We minimize the objective

$$\Phi_{tot}\left(\{\mathcal{Y}_l\}_{l=1,2,\ldots,L}\right) = \sum_{l=1}^{L} \Phi_l\left(\mathcal{Y}_l\right) + \mu \sum_{l=1}^{L-1} \Psi_{l,l+1}\left(\mathcal{Y}_l, \mathcal{Y}_{l+1}\right). \tag{2}$$

The first term enforces intra-slice embedding quality and the second term encodes the manifold alignment objective.

The intra-position embedding objective Φ quantifies distance preservation upon embedding, with all embedding derived from ambient samples of images acquired at the same location l:

$$\Phi_l\left(\mathcal{Y}_l\right) = \sum_{i}^{N} \left| \boldsymbol{Y}_{i,l} - \sum_{j \in \Omega(i)} W_{ij} \boldsymbol{Y}_{j,l} \right|^2 \tag{3}$$

Where W are the same reconstruction weights defined in 1 based on the corresponding ambient $\mathcal{X}_l$ high-dimensional neighbors. Minimizing Φ alone amounts to the standard locally linear embedding (LLE) method [8].

The inter-position objective drives the alignment of the embeddings across the submanifolds from different imaging locations.

$$\Psi_{l,l+1}\left(\mathcal{Y}_l, \mathcal{Y}_{l+1}\right) = \sum_{i_1,i_2} \left| \boldsymbol{Y}_{i_1}^{(l)} - \boldsymbol{Y}_{i_2}^{(l+1)} \right|^2 U_{i_1,i_2} \tag{4}$$

Where $\boldsymbol{Y}_l$ and $\boldsymbol{Y}_{l+1}$ are the set of embeddings corresponding to acquisitions at two different slice positions. For embeddings $\boldsymbol{Y}_{i_1}^{(l)}$ and $\boldsymbol{Y}_{i_2}^{(l+1)}$, their relevance is assessed with kernel U_{i_1,i_2}, defined as

$$U_{i_1,i_2} = exp\left(-\frac{1}{2\sigma^2} \left\| \boldsymbol{X}_{i_1}^{(l)} - \boldsymbol{X}_{i_2}^{(l+1)} \right\|_{\tilde{\mathcal{L}}_2}^2 \right) \tag{5}$$

Where σ is a kernel parameter and $\tilde{\mathcal{L}}_2$ is the normalized intensity distances.

Finally, a one-to-one correspondence across different imaging locations l is established while minimizing the matching differences [6].

When a new sample is acquired, its embedding is derived using an out-of-sample extension for LLE [8]. Specifically, reconstruction weights were derived using the K most similar training images acquired at the same spatial location from (1). Embeddings are derived by applying the same weights to the embedding vectors associated with each involved neighbor

$$\hat{Y} = \sum_{j=1}^{K} W_j \boldsymbol{Y}_j \tag{6}$$

where W_j are the weights derived from the high-dimensional images and $\boldsymbol{Y}_j$ are the out-of-sample embeddings.

2.2 Population of Motion and Contours

Similarly, the motion vector, characterized by a deformation vector field (DVF) can be propagated using the derived weights:

$$D = \sum_{j \in \Omega} W_j D_j, \tag{7}$$

where D_j are the DVFs corresponding to each nearest neighbor.

The DVFs can then be used to populate target definition in all slices. Figure 1 shows a schematic describing embedding a newly acquired 2D image in the underlying nonlinear manifold and automatically generating target contours.

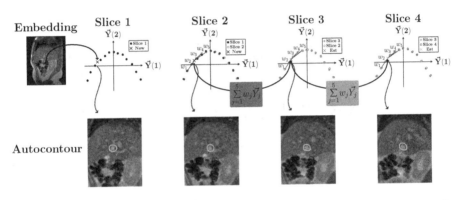

Fig. 1. The embedding process for a newly acquired image at slice 1, transferring the embedding across the aligned manifolds to all other slice positions and automatically contouring the target in the other slice positions.

In this specific implementation, we used $N = 100$ training images and neighborhood sizes of $|\Omega| = K = 25$ at each slice position to derive a embedding of dimension 3. The inter-slice parameters included a μ of 5 and σ of 1. Manifold learning was repeated to update the low dimensional embeddings using the most recent images after every 10 new images were acquired at each slice position. The images were convolved with a 6×6 averaging filter to reduce the influence of noise and cropped prior to manifold learning to avoid distraction from irrelevant state changes, such as gas in the bowel.

2.3 Target Prediction

Out-of-Sample Based Prediction. For the purpose of prediction, the state is defined as two consecutive 3D contours $S = [C_i, C_{i-1}]$, where C is the 3D binary contour and the index indicates the relative time the contour was generated.

To perform prediction at state S, we apply the out-out-sample rationale to identify similar states in the past and estimate their relevance to the current state by finding the simplex W

$$arg \min_{W} \left\| \boldsymbol{S} - \sum_{j=1}^{K} w_j \boldsymbol{S}_j \right\|^2$$

$$\text{subject to} \sum_{w_j} = 1, w_j \geq 0, j = 1, \ldots, K. \tag{8}$$

The simplex weights are then used to combine the succeeding volumes $\check{C}$'s from training set to provide an probabilistic estimate for the predicted volume, similar to an atlas-based approach. In this work, we use a simple threshold of 0.5 to generate the predicted volumetric mask estimate.

Figure 2 illustrates this coherent approach for both volumetric inference and prediction.

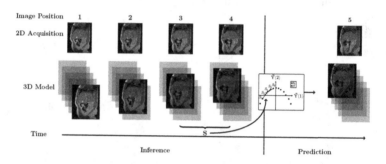

Fig. 2. Volumetric inference and prediction based on embedding.

Benchmark Prediction Methods. The proposed method was compared against four benchmark methods: a nearest neighbor prediction model derived from image similarity (IS), an autoregressive prediction method (AR), linear extrapolation (Extrapolation) and assuming the target will remain static until another image is acquired again at the same position (None).

The IS method considers two consecutive images as state $\boldsymbol{S}$, and uses only the images acquired at the same slice locations as the current images to train the prediction, using the same method as in (8) for prediction. Note that this prediction only generates a contour on a *single* slice.

The linear AR method generates prediction as a linear combination of previous motion values by minimizing

$$arg \min_{\beta} \sum_{i=1}^{N} \left| D_i - \beta_0 - \sum_{q=1}^{p} \beta_q D_{i-q} \right|^2 \tag{9}$$

where β are the fitting coefficients. The regression coefficients are then applied to the recent motion state $D_i, D_{i-1}, \ldots, D_{i-p+1}$ to generate the prediction. We used $N = 90$ samples and $p = 7$ trajectory points to fit the model. The model was updated with each newly acquired image.

Extrapolation assumes constant target velocity to extrapolate the future position from two most recent samples. Motion values acquired at the same position as the currently imaged slice were used to perform motion extrapolation.

No commercially available MRI-guided radiotherapy systems provide the option to perform motion prediction. The target is implicitly assumed to be static until the next image is acquired. The "None" benchmark reflects this behavior.

3   Method

3.1   Studies and Evaluation

A total of eight healthy volunteers were recruited to evaluate the proposed method. Images were acquired repeatedly in an interleaved fashion across 10 slice positions using a 0.35 T MRI-guided radiotherapy system. Images were acquired at approximately 3 frames per second until 200 images were acquired at each slice position using a balanced steady state free precession sequence with a $2 \times 2\,mm^2$ in-plane resolution and 4.5 mm slice thickness. All predictions were performed one image frame (0.33 s) into the future, which falls into the range of 200–500 ms [5] system latency for MRI-guided radiotherapy systems. Normal anatomical features were contoured on the reference image at each slice location. All motion vector fields were derived using a 2D multi-resolution B-Spline based deformable registration to a reference image of the same slice location to enable contour generation [4].

Since at the imaging frequency of 3 Hz we only have access to a single 2D image slice at one of the 10 slice locations, there is no access to the ground-truth volumetric target definition. Quantitative evaluation was performed by retrospectively evaluating the intersection between the target volume prediction and the ground-truth image at the specific slice where the image was acquired. Dice similarity coefficient (DSC) and contour distance were used as performance metrics. A t-test was used to compare performance between the proposed method and the benchmark approaches. We call this "conditional 2D performance" to differentiate it from a truly 3D assessment.

The proposed embedding approach is the only method that generated volumetric predictions. To evaluate the performance of the 3D prediction, the dice similarity was compared between the predicted and retrospectively inferred 3D contour volume generated by the embedding approach, referred to as the "3D performance" quantification.

3.2   Results

Examination of the conditional 2D performance shows that the proposed prediction method resulted in an average dice similarity of 0.84 and mean centroid prediction error of 1.74 mm across all healthy volunteer studies. Figure 3 reports comparison of the proposed method to the benchmarks for these two metrics.

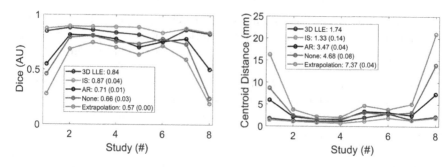

Fig. 3. Performance comparison in DSC and centroid distance prediction error for each healthy volunteer study. The average result and the companion p-value from t-test (in bracket) are reported.

In the conditional 2D performance assessment, the IS method performs best. The proposed 3D method comes in a close second, possibly due to the smoothing introduced in embedding and manifold alignment. In the 3D performance assessment, the proposed method achieves an average DSC of 0.87. Table 1 reports the mean and standard deviation of DSC for each subject.

Table 1. The average and standard deviation of the dice similarity between the 3D predicted and 3D observed target contours for each healthy volunteer study along with the in-plane target area

Volunteer	1	2	3	4	5	6	7	8
Average	0.89	0.92	0.89	0.86	0.84	0.80	0.89	0.84
Standard deviation	0.13	0.07	0.09	0.11	0.15	0.14	0.08	0.14
In-plane target area (mm²)	1144	1080	632	452	1076	1584	1656	1364

4 Discussions and Outlook

We have demonstrated the proposed method of simultaneous manifold embedding and alignment can be used to provide complete volumetric target predictions in real-time during MRI-guided radiotherapy for treatment guidance. Importantly, the proposed method provides 3D target contours in a unified geometrical space at the native 2D image acquisition frame rate, bridging the gap between the desire to drive treatment decisions using full 3D information and limited imaging speed.

In the conditional 2D assessment, the proposed method comes as a close second to the IS prediction, and outperforms all other benchmarks investigated. The reduction in prediction performance compared to the IS method may be attributable to the smoothing during embedding and alignment, and could possibly be addressed with further investigation of embedding parameters. Additionally, the proposed method derives prediction weights from the 3D binary target masks whereas the IS method derives prediction weights from image similarity. It is possible that either texture within the target, the surrounding context, or both may help inform prediction. The proposed approach is amicable to such modifications by changing the definition of state to ROI-intensity. All other benchmarks rely upon repeated sampling of the same motion information at the same spatial location, resulting in a long effective look-ahead length that was 10 times the imaging interval under the interleaved acquisition protocol.

The proposed prediction performance was lowest in volunteer study 6. This particular volunteer's breathing motion was irregular as the subject changed their way of breathing, switching between chest and abdominal breathing during the recording. This type of switching poses challenges for the IS method as well, though not as severe. It is possible to expand the current method to a hybrid scheme by incorporating a pattern change detection module to adapt the estimation of the underlying manifold more rapidly once a switching behavior is identified.

Finally, our method was motivated by the interleaved image acquisition in MRI guided radiotherapy, to utilize 2D images of varying slice location as input and provide real-time 3D volumetric characterization as output. The same rationale applies to other scenarios where partial, limited observation is acquired online, such as in fluoroscopic settings for adaptive radiotherapy.

References

1. Baumgartner, C.F., Kolbitsch, C., McClelland, J.R., Rueckert, D., King, A.P.: Autoadaptive motion modelling for MR-based respiratory motion estimation. Med. Image Anal. **35**, 83–100 (2017)
2. Ginn, J.S., Ruan, D., Low, D.A., Lamb, J.M.: Multislice motion modeling for MRI-guided radiotherapy gating. Med. Phys. **46**(2), 465–474 (2019)
3. Harris, W., Ren, L., Cai, J., Zhang, Y., Chang, Z., Yin, F.F.: A technique for generating volumetric cine-magnetic resonance imaging. Int. J. Radiat. Oncol.* Biol.* Phys. **95**(2), 844–853 (2016)
4. Klein, S., Staring, M., Murphy, K., Viergever, M.A., Pluim, J.P., et al.: Elastix: a toolbox for intensity-based medical image registration. IEEE Trans. Med. Imaging **29**(1), 196 (2010)
5. Lamb, J.M., et al.: Dosimetric validation of a magnetic resonance image gated radiotherapy system using a motion phantom and radiochromic film. J. Appl. Clin. Med. Phys. **18**(3), 163–169 (2017)
6. Munkres, J.: Algorithms for the assignment and transportation problems. J. Soc. Ind. Appl. Math. **5**(1), 32–38 (1957)
7. Noorda, Y.H., Bartels, L.W., Viergever, M.A., Pluim, J.P.: Subject-specific liver motion modeling in MRI: a feasibility study on spatiotemporal prediction. Phys. Med. Biol. **62**(7), 2581 (2017)
8. Saul, L.K., Roweis, S.T.: Think globally, fit locally: unsupervised learning of low dimensional manifolds. J. Mach. Learn. Res. **4**(Jun), 119–155 (2003)
9. Seregni, M., et al.: Motion prediction in MRI-guided radiotherapy based on interleaved orthogonal cine-MRI. Phys. Med. Biol. **61**(2), 872 (2016)

One-Dimensional Convolutional Network for Dosimetry Evaluation at Organs-at-Risk in Esophageal Radiation Treatment Planning

Dashan Jiang[1], Teng Li[1(✉)], Ronghu Mao[2], Chi Du[3], Yongbin Liu[1], Shuolin Liu[1], and Jianfei Liu[1]

[1] Electrical Engineering and Automation, Anhui University, Hefei, China
`tenglwy@gmail.com`
[2] Radiation Oncology, The Affiliated Cancer Hospital of Zhengzhou University, Zhengzhou, China
[3] Cancer Center, The Second Peoples Hospital of Neijiang, Neijiang, Sichuan, China

Abstract. Dose volume histogram (DVH) is an important dosimetry evaluation metric and it plays an important role in guiding the development of esophageal ra-diotherapy treatment plans. Automatic DVH prediction is therefore very use-ful to achieve high-quality esophageal treatment planning. This paper studied stacked denoise auto-encoder (SDAE) to compute correlation between DVH and distance to target histogram (DTH) based on the fact that the geometric information between PTV and OAR is closely related to DVH, this study aims to establish a multi-OAR geometry-dosimetry model through deep learning to achieve DVH prediction. Distance to target histogram (DTH) is chosen to measure the geometrical relationship between PTV and OARs. In the proposed method, stacked denoise auto-encoder (SDAE) is used to reduce the dimension of the extracted DTH and DVH features, and then one-dimensional convolutional network (one-DCN) is used for the correlation modeling. This model can predict the DVH of multiple OARs based on the individual patient's geometry without manual removal of radiation plans with outliers. The average prediction error of the measurement focusing on the left lung, right lung, heart, spinal cord was less than 5%. The predicted DVHs could thus provide accurate optimization parameters, which could be a useful reference for physicists to reduce planning time.

Keywords: Esophagus · Dose volume histogram · Stacked denoise auto-encoder · One-dimensional convolutional network

This work is supported by the National Natural Science Foundation of China (No. 61702001), and the Anhui Provincial Natural Science Foundation of China (No. 1908085J25), and Key Support Program of University Outstanding Youth Talent of Anhui Province (No. gxyqZD2018007), and Open fund for Discipline Construction, Institute of Physical Science and Information Technology, Anhui University.

D. Nguyen et al. (Eds.): AIRT 2019, LNCS 11850, pp. 86–93, 2019.
https://doi.org/10.1007/978-3-030-32486-5_11

1   Introduction

Radiotherapy treatment planning is a complicated process, which attempts to compromise the high dosage delivery at the planned target volume while minimizing dosing amount at organs-at-risk (OARs) [1]. To achieve this goal, the dose-volume histogram (DVH) is often used to guide the physicists to manually adjust the cumbersome parameters. Therefore, DVH prediction would be clinically useful for treatment plan design, which is empirically proved to be highly cor-related with the distance between OARs and PTVs. Modeling DVHs with the geometrical distance between PTVs and OARs is thus the main theme in this work.

In recent years, many research teams have used knowledge-based planning (KBP) to model such correlation. Distance to target histogram (DTH) was utilized by Zhu et al. [2] to represent the geometrical relationship by computing the volume fraction of an OAR controlled by different distances to PTV. The correlation between DTH and DVH was modeled by principal component analysis (PCA) and linear regression. Yuan [3] extensively explored different types of features to describe the geometrical relationship and systematically analyzed their correlation with DVH. Deep belief network (DBN) was used to model the correlation between DTH and DVH after dimensional reduction by auto-encoder [4]. However, due to the existence of the anisotropy of radiotherapy plans, outliers in the data also become one of the factors affecting the accuracy of the predicted DVH model [5]. The common auto-encoder cannot avoid the effects of outliers, and the ability to fit nonlinearities of DBN is not as good as that of convolutional networks.

The development of deep learning [6] in recent years has opens a new avenue to compute correlation, which is the main scope of this paper. In this paper, stack denoise auto-encoder (SDAE) [7] is utilized to reduce the feature dimension for DVH and DTH, and one-dimensional convolution network (one-DCN) is then adapted to model their correlation. Such correlation can be used to predict DVH for new patients. Validation results showed that the predicted and clinical DVHs were close to each other, and the predicted model has a significant robustness to the outliers of the data, which can significantly reduce the planning time by predicting the DVH to quickly approach the near-optimal parameter settings.

2   Methods and Materials

Figure 1 depictures the proposed framework. First, the CT image and the required structural contour image, that is, the structure of PTV and each OAR, are extracted from the original data of the DICOM data format. Next, it included of a modeling process (solid frame) that compute the correlation between DTH and DVH and a prediction process (dashed frame) that exploits the correlation model to predict DVH for new patients. Both processes contain data preprocess to ex-tract the geometrical relationship between PTV and OARs, stack denoise auto-encoder to reduce feature dimension, and one-dimensional convolution network to model the correlation.

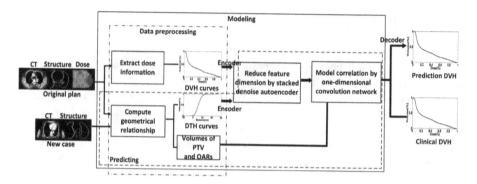

Fig. 1. The proposed framework contains a modeling process (solid frame) that computes the correlation between DVH and DTH and a prediction process (dashed frame) that predicts DVH based on the modeled correlation. Both processes involve three main steps: (1) data preprocessing to compute dose information (DVH) and geometrical information (DTH), respectively, (2) stack denoise auto-encoder to reduce feature dimension, and (3) one-dimensional convolution network to model the correlation.

2.1 Patient Data

We collected 182 intensity-modulated radiation therapy (IMRT) esophageal plans and 88 volume modulated arc therapy (VMAT) esophageal plans. All IMRT plans share the same configuration of seven-field 6 MV photon beams, with the gantry angles at 135°, 165°, 195°, 0°, 30°, 225°, and 330°. The prescription dose (Rx = 78 Gy) covers at least 95% of the PTV volume. And selected VMAT plans used two 6MV coplanar arcs with a prescription dose of 61.02 Gy. We only predicted left lung, left lung, heart, and spine cord in this study.

2.2 Data Preprocessing

This step aims to develop a feature descriptor to describe the geometrical relationship between PTV and OARs. An array of geometric features was analyzed to study their contributions to OAR dose sparing. In an esophageal radiation treatment plan, PTV and OAR contours are put in structure images, as illustrated in the top images of Fig. 1. We use DTH to measure the geometrical relationship among all these contours. DTH refer to cumulative OAR volumes within a certain distance from the PTV surface. Specifically, DTH can be defined as:

$$DTH(r) = \frac{|V_{OAR}^r \cap V_{PTV}|}{|V_{OAR}|} \tag{1}$$

Where V_{OAR} and V_{PTV} represent the voxel sets of OAR and PTV, respectively. V_{OAR}^r represents the voxel sets of OAR with a maximum distance r from the surface of the PTV. Where r is the Euclidean form of the distance function $r(V_{OAR}^i, PTV)$ from the OAR voxel to the PTV surface. Supposing S_{PTV} be the set of surface points in PTV, the distance between an OAR voxel V_{OAR}^i to the PTV is given by

$$r(V_{OAR}^i, PTV) = min_k \left\{ \left\| V_{OAR}^i - V_{PTV}^k \right\| \qquad |V_{PTV}^k \in S_{PTV} \right\} \qquad (2)$$

Negative $r(V_{OAR}^i, PTV)$ indicates that the voxel V_{OAR} is inside the PTV boundary and positive means outside. So intuitively, the meaning of DTH is the OAR voxel at a certain distance from the surface boundary of the PTV.

In this study, we select 50 points with equal spacing from the DTH curve as a discretized high-dimensional representation of the distance-dose continuous function curve. Each point contains a volume fraction value and a distance value. We hold all the discrete distance values and only select the corresponding volume score values to construct a 50-dimensional DTH feature vector. In the modeling process, we also compute DVH based on the dose values received by the corresponding OAR in the dose image. Another 50-dimensional DVH feature vector can be constructed by combining dose values of 50 points in the DVH curve.

2.3 Feature Dimension Reduction by Stacked Denoise Auto-encoder

DTH and DVH feature vectors from the previous step often contain noise, and high dimensional feature vectors also leverage the computational cost. So the purpose of this step is to extract the main components of DVH and DTH from multiple OARs.

In previous research work, principal component analysis (PCA) often used as a common dimensionality reduction method to reduce the DTH and DVH feature vectors. Nevertheless, PCA also has some drawbacks. For example, PCA only performs well if the sample distribution obeys the standard gaussian distribution, and the existence of outliers often leads to the inapplicability of PCA. Self-supervised neural networks usually perform better for nonlinear dimensionality reduction. Self-supervised layer-by-layer training makes more attention to the feature distribution of the original data in the dimension reduction process, while avoiding the gradient disappearance caused by back propagation (BP). Therefore, auto-encoder (SDAE) is used to nonlinear reduction of dimension and principal component extraction in our work.

SDAE is a self-supervised learning method. By adding noise into the original data and layer-by-layer unsupervised learning, SDAE effectively achieves the dimensionality reduction. The SDAE contains eight encoding layers (64-128-256-128-64-32-16-5) and eight decoding layers (16-32-64-128-256-128-64-50). As shown in Fig. 2, encoder and decoder are structurally symmetric, the random noise is subject to a Gaussian distribution and matches the original data dimension.

It should be noted that unlike the DVH distribution, the difference in the discrete distribution of the start and end of all DTH distributions is very small, so the gaussian kernel function is assigned to the loss function to weigh each sampling point when fine-tuning SDAE. This approach allows the network to

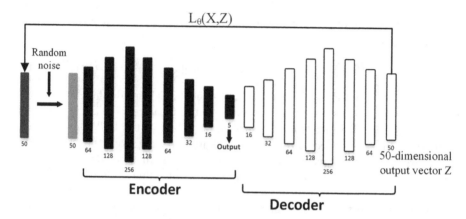

Fig. 2. Overview of the SDAE structure for reducing DVH and DTH feature vector dimensions. The SDAE contains eight encoding layers and eight decoding layers. Here, the blue box represents the original input 50-dimensional feature vector, the gray box represents the 50-dimensional feature vector with the random noise, the coding layer is shown in black boxes, and the decoding layer is shown in white boxes. The number below the box represents the number of neurons in each layer, and $L_\theta(X, Z)$ represents the loss function between the reconstructed feature vector and the original input feature vector. (Color figure online)

better capture the important features of the DTH curve, that is, the part with the largest change rate in DTH curves. The improved loss function is similar to the local weighted regression loss function, which is given by

$$L(\theta) = \sum_{i=1}^{m} w^i (h_\theta(x^i) - x^i)^2 \tag{3}$$

Where x represents one of the elements of the input feature vector, and m is total the number of neurons in the feature vector. $h_\theta(x^i)$ indicates that the i-th neuron has been reconstructed by SDAE. The weight w^i here obeys the standard gaussian distribution. According to experience, the mean value of this distribution is generally located at the median point of 50 sampling points due to the rate of change of DTH curves here is the largest.

By layer-by-layer pre-training of each layer, the SDAE can gradually reduce a 50-dimensional feature vector either from DVH or DTH into a 5-dimensional one, Here, 5-dimensional output feature was empirically determined because it only has less than 3% information loss from the original input.

2.4   Correlation Modelling Using One-Dimensional Convolution Network

According to Yuan's study, dosimetric goals of one OAR dose sparing is affected by multi-OAR geometries. This step exploits the reduced feature vectors from the

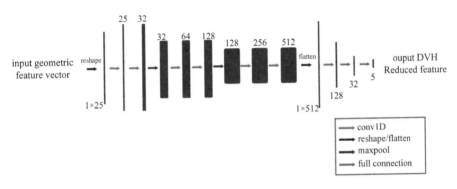

Fig. 3. Overview of the one-DCN structure. Each blue box represents a multi-channel feature vector, and channel number is put on its top. The Feature vector size is list at the lower left edge of each box. Arrows denote different operations, and their meanings are put in the legend. (Color figure online)

previous step to nonlinearly model the correlation between multi-OAR geometric features and DVH. The one-dimensional convolutional network (one-DCN) can extract the translation features of one-dimensional data better than the traditional regression method or the common neural network (such as DBN). Therefore, one-DCN is adopted to model the nonlinear correlation between geometric features and DVH. As shown in Fig. 3, small (3×3) convolution filters were used in all layers, and all convolution layers are equipped with the rectification (ReLU) non-linearity. An L2-regularization term and a smoothing term are added to the objective function in ONE-DCN model. The final regularized solution objective function can be expressed as Eq. (4):

$$W = argmin_\theta \left\{ \|F(X|W) - Y\|_2^2 + \lambda_1 \|W\|_2^2 + \lambda_2 \|\triangledown W\|_2^2 \right\} \tag{4}$$

Where $F(X|W)$ represents the output feature vector computed by the input feature vector X through the one-DCN model. $\lambda_1 \|W\|_2^2$ represents the L2-regularization term, and $\lambda_2 \|\triangledown W\|_2^2$ represents an additional smoothing regularization term which can ensure that contributions from adjacent DTH reduced dimension components within one OAR to the DVH components vary smoothly.

In this experiment, the geometric features include all OAR and PTV volume feature vectors and each reduced to a 5-dimensional DTH feature vector of one OAR by the SDAE. Accordingly, the dose features include reduction to a 5-dimensional DVH feature vector by the SDAE. Note that each ONE-DCN model here corresponds to an OAR DVH prediction.

When predicting DVH for an OAR from new patients, the DTH of the OAR is first computed. A 50-dimensional DTH feature vector can be established by sampling DTH curve and this feature vector is then reduced to a 5-dimensional feature vector by the SDAE. Its corresponding 5-dimensional DVH feature vector can be reconstructed in terms of the established ONE-DCN model. Finally, we can use the decoding layers in the SDAE to reconstruct a DVH feature vector, which can be used to predict DVH for the current OAR. Therefore, we can use the same procedure to model and predict DVHs of all OARs for esophageal patients.

3 Results

Table 1 show the mean error values of the dose endpoint values for the left lung and spinal cord of the two models for predicting DVH, in two different experiments, respectively. From the quantitative average error analysis in Table 1, the proposed prediction model is compared with the traditional prediction model, the proposed prediction model has stronger robustness ($p = 0.012$) and better prediction effect ($p < 0.001$) under different outlier environments.

The comparison of DVHs for a subset of the validation plans are shown in Fig. 4. The figure shows that all OAR DVH curves can be achieved by the proposed model to achieve a better prediction. The experiment results mean that the proposed model can accurately predict DVH and provide near-optimal parameters to reduce manual parameter adjustment in radiation treatment planning.

Table 1. Average prediction volume fractions errors of the left lung and right lung between predicted and clinical DVHs at 5% (V5), 10% (v10), 20% (v20), and 30% (v30) prescription dose.

OARs	Methods	Dose Endpoint error (Left Lung)			
		V5	V10	V20	V30
Left lung	PCA+SVR	$5.9 \pm 3.5\%$	$7.84 \pm 4.1\%$	$6.86 \pm 5.7\%$	$6.43 \pm 4.8\%$
Left lung	SDAE+one-DCN	$2.33 \pm 1.2\%$	$2.68 \pm 2.8\%$	$3.45 \pm 2.7\%$	$2.91 \pm 3.3\%$
Right lung	PCA+SVR	$2.69 \pm 1.8\%$	$5.12 \pm 3.7\%$	$4.36 \pm 1.9\%$	$5.81 \pm 3.6\%$
Right lung	SDAE+one-DCN	$2.02 \pm 0.9\%$	$3.27 \pm 1.3\%$	$4.53 \pm 1.5\%$	$3.02 \pm 2.7\%$

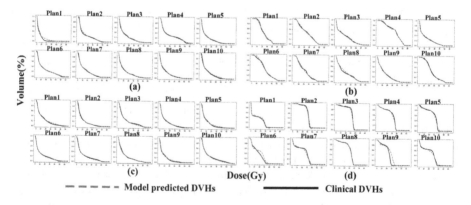

Fig. 4. Comparison of predicted and clinical DVHs of left lung (a), right lung (b), heart (c), and spine cord (d) using the proposed model. the solid black line indicates the DVH in the esophageal radiotherapy clinical plan, and the red dotted line indicates the DVH generated by the model prediction.

4   Conclusion

We developed a model to automatically predict dose volume histograms at OARs based on their geometrical relationship with PTV for esophageal radiation treatment planning. This model is designed for reaching a personalized treatment goal by (1) Time-consuming optimization of artificial optimization parameters (2) The traditional prediction model is not robust to environmental performance with outliers. Such a model can be used to predict DVHs of different OARs for new patients. Experiments show that our model has strong robustness and high prediction accuracy under different outlier environments. The average prediction error of the measurement focus of the left lung, right lung, heart, spinal cord is not higher than 5%. Accurate DVH prediction can provide near-optimal parameters for esophageal treatment planning, which can significantly reduce the planning time. In the future, we are planning to expand our predicted model to simultaneously predict DVHs for all OARs instead of predicting them sequentially in this work.

References

1. Nelms, B.E., et al.: Variation in external beam treatment plan quality: an interinstitutional study of planners and planning systems. Pract. Radiat. Oncol. **2**, 296–305 (2012)
2. Xiaofeng, Z., Yaorong, G., Taoran, L., Danthai, T., Fang-Fang, Y., Jackie, W.Q.: A planning quality evaluation tool for prostate adaptive IMRT based on machine learning. Med. Phys. **38**(2), 719 (2011)
3. Yuan, L., Ge, Y., Lee, W.R., Yin, F.F., Kirkpatrick, J.P., Wu, Q.J.: Quantitative analysis of the factors which affect the interpatient organ-at-risk dose sparing variation in IMRT plans. Med. Phys. **39**(11), 6868–6878 (2012)
4. Jiang, D., Li, T., Mao, R., et al.: Deep belief network for dosimetry evaluation at organs-at-risk in esophageal radiation treatment planning. In: Basic & Clinical Pharmacology & Toxicology, vol. 124, pp. 224–225. Wiley, NJ USA (2019)
5. Delaney, A.R., Tol, J.P., Dahele, M., Cuijpers, J., Slotman, B.J., Verbakel, W.F.A.R.: Effect of do-simetric outliers on the performance of a commercial knowledge-based planning solution. Int. J. Radiat. Oncol. Biol. Phys. **94**(3), 469–77 (2016)
6. Lecun, Y., Bengio, Y., Hinton, G.: Deep learning. Nature **521**(7553), 436 (2015)
7. Bengio, Y., Lamblin, P., Popovici, D., et al.: Greedy layer-wise training of deep networks. Adv. Neural Inf. Process. Syst. **19**, 153–160 (2007)

Unpaired Synthetic Image Generation in Radiology Using GANs

Denis Prokopenko[1,2]([✉]) [iD], Joël Valentin Stadelmann[2], Heinrich Schulz[3],
Steffen Renisch[3], and Dmitry V. Dylov[1] [iD]

[1] Skolkovo Institute of Science and Technology, Moscow, Russian Federation
{denis.prokopenko,d.dylov}@skoltech.ru
[2] Philips Innovation Labs RUS, Moscow, Russian Federation
joel.stadelmann@philips.com
[3] Philips GmbH Innovative Technologies, Hamburg, Germany
{heinrich.schulz,steffen.renisch}@philips.com

Abstract. In this work, we investigate approaches to generating synthetic Computed Tomography (CT) images from the real Magnetic Resonance Imaging (MRI) data. Generating the radiological scans has grown in popularity in the recent years due to its promise to enable single-modality radiotherapy planning in clinical oncology, where the co-registration of the radiological modalities is cumbersome. We rely on the Generative Adversarial Network (GAN) models with cycle consistency which permit unpaired image-to-image translation between the modalities. We also introduce the perceptual loss function term and the coordinate convolutional layer to further enhance the quality of translated images. The Unsharp masking and the Super-Resolution GAN (SRGAN) were considered to improve the quality of synthetic images. The proposed architectures were trained on the unpaired MRI-CT data and then evaluated on the paired brain dataset. The resulting CT scans were generated with the mean absolute error (MAE), the peak signal-to-noise ratio (PSNR) and the structural similarity (SSIM) scores of 60.83 HU, 17.21 dB, and 0.8, respectively. DualGAN with perceptual loss function term and coordinate convolutional layer proved to perform best. The MRI-CT translation approach holds potential to eliminate the need for the patients to undergo both examinations and to be clinically accepted as a new tool for radiotherapy planning.

Keywords: Deep learning · Image translation · Radiotherapy

1 Introduction

Cancer is one of the major causes of death across the Globe [15]. In 50% of hospitalisations related to oncology, the patients are prescribed radiation therapy [6], the goal of which is to destroy the malignant neoplasms. Ionising radiation is delivered to a patient according to a dose plan derived from MRI and CT examinations [4]. The MRI is used to locate the tumour with high fidelity thanks to

© Springer Nature Switzerland AG 2019
D. Nguyen et al. (Eds.): AIRT 2019, LNCS 11850, pp. 94–101, 2019.
https://doi.org/10.1007/978-3-030-32486-5_12

its superior soft-tissue contrast [10], whereas the CT scan effectively measures the density of the tissues and determines the dose of necessary radiation [1].

Prior to radiotherapy, a patient has to undergo two different imaging procedures in two different scanners. This always leads to a misplacement of the body position, to large shifting errors, and to a misalignment of the targeted organs on the MRI and CT images. Consequently, an inadequate calculation of a radiation dose frequently occurs [2]. Carrying out both procedures also involves extra financial burden and extra X-ray radiation exposure in the CT machine.

The MRI-only radiotherapy approach can eliminate the aforementioned disadvantages [9]. The radiotherapy plan can instead be derived from the MRI scan combined with a perfectly co-aligned synthetic CT volume generated from the MRI itself. As a result, the patient can skip the CT examination.

In this work we focus on MRI-to-CT image translation by CNNs. Zhu et al. [24] introduced the CycleGAN with cycle consistency to address the unpaired aspect of the image-to-image translation problem. Each half of the cycle translates an image from one domain to the other, while the whole cycle performs the image translation to the initial domain. The approach was directly applied to MRI-CT image translation by Wolterink et al. [21]. Yi et al. [22] proposed a similar DualGAN model with the cycle consistency and more flexible cycle loss function (see Eq. 1 below).

Liu et al. [13] proposed unsupervised image-to-image translation network (UNIT) with a similar idea of translation between two domains. The UNIT model takes advantage of cycle consistency as well, but the translation is done via a shared latent invariant space, where images from the both domains have identical representations.

Zhang et al. [23] proposed HarmonicGAN that bidirectionally translates images between the source and the target domains. Its objective is also built on the cycle consistency, but it was upgraded with smooth regularisation.

Here, we study the cycle consistency architecture with perceptual loss function term [8] and coordinate convolutional layer [7,14,17]. In addition, we report application of Super-Resolution GAN [11] and Unsharp masking [16] filters to improve both the training and the generated images.

2   Methods

In this work, we chose DualGAN [22] as a baseline in application to MRI-CT image translation. The perceptual loss function term [8] and coordinate convolutional layer [14] were embedded to DualGAN to improve the quality of the translation. The SRGAN [11] and Unsharp masking [16] were incorporated to pipeline as image post-processing and pre-processing methods.

The DualGAN architecture [22] consists of two image generators and two patch discriminators, see Fig. 1. The first generator $G_{MRI \to CT}$ is trained to translate an MRI scan I_{MRI} to CT image $G_{MRI \to CT}(I_{MRI})$; the second generator $G_{CT \to MRI}$ translates image from a CT domain I_{CT} to MRI image $G_{CT \to MRI}(I_{CT})$. These two generators form a cycle, which allows comparing

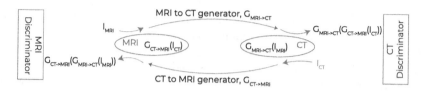

Fig. 1. DualGAN architecture.

the reconstructed image with the original. The cycle loss function (1) consists of two terms, which are mean absolute errors between MRI image and MRI reconstruction and between CT image and CT reconstruction, respectively, with adjustable parameters λ_{MRI} and λ_{CT}.

$$\mathcal{L}_{cyc} = \lambda_{MRI} \|G_{CT \to MRI}(G_{MRI \to CT}(I_{MRI})) - I_{MRI}\|_1 \\ + \lambda_{CT} \|G_{MRI \to CT}(G_{CT \to MRI}(I_{CT})) - I_{CT}\|_1 \tag{1}$$

The patch discriminators distinguish generated images from real ones. They force generators to perform more realistic translation. The output of each discriminator estimates the realness of the input image, which is used in learning as an adversarial term (2) with an adjustable parameter of λ_D.

$$-\lambda_D \Big(\log \big(D_{CT} \left(G_{MRI \to CT} \left(I_{MRI} \right) \right) \big) + \log \big(D_{MRI} \left(G_{CT \to MRI} \left(I_{CT} \right) \right) \big) \Big) \tag{2}$$

The perceptual loss function was introduced as a part of super-resolution problem and style transfer problem [8]. The objective builds on the idea of feature matching: high-level representations of two images are compared by mean squared error. The pre-trained VGG-16 model provides high-level representations - the outputs of the intermediate level, see Fig. 2. Although VGG-16 is not optimised for tomographic images, its use is still relevant: the features are extracted in an identical way for both images. The result of the comparison makes loss function more sensitive to an image context leading to a more realistic image generation.

The coordinate convolutional layer was proposed by Liu et al. [14] to take into account spatial information of the image. Two additional slices with i and j coordinates are concatenated with the tensor representation of the image,

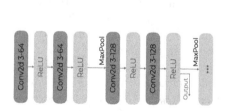

Fig. 2. 8th output of VGG-16.

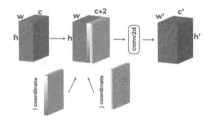

Fig. 3. Coordinate convolutional layer.

see Fig. 3. The new tensor with coordinates is passed to the usual convolutional layer. The coordinate convolutional layer helps to distinguish black pixels of MRI T1-weighted images, which could represent either a bone or air.

Super-Resolution GAN and **Unsharp masking** were used to improve the quality of image appearance. Super-Resolution GAN is capable of inferring photo-realistic natural images with 4x upscaling factor [11]. Unsharp masking enables creating sharp images combining negative blurred images with the original ones [16]. SRGAN and Unsharp were applied as post-processing for synthetic images generated by considered architectures, and as pre-processing before training.

3   Data

Three medical datasets were obtained to work with the considered methods of unpaired MRI to CT translation.

MRI T1-weighted volumes of 7 patients were obtained from CPTAC Phase 3 dataset [3,5]. CT volumes of 61 patients were used from Head-and-neck cancer dataset [19,20]. The private dataset consists of paired CT, MRI T1-weighted and mask volumes of 10 patients.

The MRI images were initially pre-processed. The initial pixel values were linearly scaled to $[0, 1]$ range. The CT scans were clipped from the $[-1000, 3000]$ HU range to a narrower $[-155, 295]$ HU. New range was linearly scaled to $[0, 1]$.

All models were trained on CPTAC/Head-and-neck sets and the training part of the private dataset. The qualitative and quantitative results were obtained on the test part of the private dataset.

4   Experiments

In this work, four different architectures were considered: DualGAN, DualGAN with the coordinate convolutional layer (DualGAN, CC), DualGAN with perceptual loss function term (DualGAN, VGG) and DualGAN with perceptual loss function term and coordinate convolutional layer (DualGAN, VGG, CC). The synthetic MRI or CT images were compared with original paired scans from the private dataset. Besides, outputs from pre-trained DualGAN and DualGAN with perceptual loss function term and coordinate convolutional layer generators were enhanced by SRGAN or Unsharp masking to obtain better quality. The same two models were trained from scratch on training data enhanced by SRGAN or Unsharp masking.

The DualGAN with perceptual loss function term and DualGAN with coordinate convolutional layer resulted in decreased quality of translation, see Table 1. However, the configuration, which combines both upgrades, outperformed the others. The MAE dropped to 60.83 HU; PSNR and SSIM rose up to 17.21 dB and 0.8 respectively. The comparison with original CT scans in the full range of HU resulted in MAE: 182.07 ± 20.17 HU, PSNR: 16.40 ± 0.51 dB, and SSIM: 0.79 ± 0.02.

Table 1. Performance comparison of different translation configurations.

Configuration	MAE, HU ↓	PSNR, dB ↑	SSIM ↑
Synthetic CT image generation			
DualGAN	62.95 ± 1.17	16.82 ± 0.83	0.79 ± 0.02
DualGAN, CC	63.27 ± 2.00	16.96 ± 0.71	0.78 ± 0.03
DualGAN, VGG	66.52 ± 3.74	16.74 ± 1.08	0.78 ± 0.03
DualGAN, VGG, CC	60.83 ± 2.20	17.21 ± 1.00	0.80 ± 0.03
Synthetic MRI image generation			
DualGAN	45.70 ± 1.71	21.98 ± 0.51	0.76 ± 0.04
DualGAN, CC	40.04 ± 2.52	22.91 ± 0.48	0.77 ± 0.03
DualGAN, VGG	42.11 ± 2.15	22.37 ± 0.59	0.77 ± 0.03
DualGAN, VGG, CC	37.99 ± 4.92	23.31 ± 0.19	0.78 ± 0.03

Even though the main purpose of the network was to generate synthetic CT images; the architecture allows generating synthetic MRI images too. The combination with both improvements surpassed other models with MAE, PSNR and SSIM equal $37.99, 23.31$ dB and 0.78 respectively.

Qualitative results are presented in Figs. 4 and 5. The considered methods can create MRI and CT images retaining the right form and shape of a head and the inner brain structure. The models can partly distinguish the air and bone pixels, the borders between other different types of tissues are shifted and blurred. The worst results concentrate on the complex structures of the nose and jaw parts.

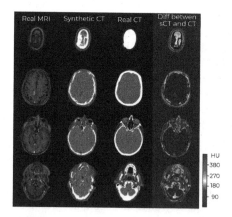

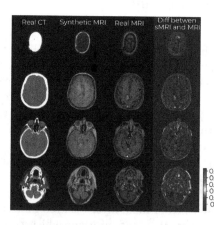

Fig. 4. Synthetic CT image generation by DualGAN, VGG, CC.

Fig. 5. Synthetic MRI image generation by DualGAN, VGG, CC.

Figures 6 and 7 show the results of SRGAN and Unsharp masking applications in relation to the DualGAN baseline. The Unsharp masking was performed by Gaussian blur with σ of $\{1, 2, 5, 10, 20\}$ and kernel size of 9. Pre-trained SRGAN [18] was used with a 4x upscale factor. The considered variations led to worse quality of generated synthetic images comparing to corresponding initial results of the DualGAN and DualGAN, VGG, CC architectures. The DualGAN, VGG, CC architecture creates the highest quality synthetic images than the same configurations with additional image enhancement, see Tables 2 and 3. We suppose that SRGAN specifically trained for MRI and CT images could lead to the greater quality of generated tomographic images.

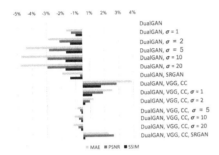

Fig. 6. Comparison of methods to post-process sCT.

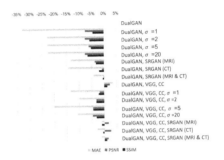

Fig. 7. Comparison of methods to pre-process training data. CT generation.

Table 2. Performance comparison of configurations with post-processing.

Configuration	MAE, HU ↓	PSNR, dB ↑	SSIM ↑
Synthetic CT image generation, post-processing case			
DualGAN	62.95 ± 1.17	16.82 ± 0.83	0.79 ± 0.02
DualGAN, $\sigma = 1$	63.63 ± 1.11	16.69 ± 0.81	0.79 ± 0.02
DualGAN, $\sigma = 2$	64.46 ± 1.29	16.55 ± 0.80	0.78 ± 0.02
DualGAN, $\sigma = 5$	65.43 ± 1.45	16.43 ± 0.80	0.78 ± 0.02
DualGAN, $\sigma = 10$	65.67 ± 1.53	16.41 ± 0.79	0.78 ± 0.02
DualGAN, $\sigma = 20$	65.68 ± 1.50	16.41 ± 0.79	0.78 ± 0.02
DualGAN with SRGAN	63.85 ± 1.17	16.80 ± 0.81	0.78 ± 0.02
DualGAN, VGG, CC	60.83 ± 2.20	17.21 ± 1.00	0.80 ± 0.03
DualGAN, VGG, CC, $\sigma = 1$	61.69 ± 2.03	17.06 ± 0.98	0.79 ± 0.03
DualGAN, VGG, CC, $\sigma = 2$	62.51 ± 1.85	16.90 ± 0.96	0.79 ± 0.03
DualGAN, VGG, CC, $\sigma = 5$	63.20 ± 1.67	16.79 ± 0.96	0.79 ± 0.03
DualGAN, VGG, CC, $\sigma = 10$	63.35 ± 1.62	16.77 ± 0.96	0.79 ± 0.03
DualGAN, VGG, CC, $\sigma = 20$	63.38 ± 1.60	16.77 ± 0.95	0.79 ± 0.03
DualGAN, VGG, CC, SRGAN	61.87 ± 2.18	17.18 ± 0.98	0.79 ± 0.03

Table 3. Performance comparison of configurations with pre-processing.

Configuration	MAE, HU ↓	PSNR, dB ↑	SSIM ↑
Synthetic CT image generation, pre-processing case			
DualGAN	62.95 ± 1.17	16.82 ± 0.83	0.79 ± 0.02
DualGAN, $\sigma = 1$	83.62 ± 8.13	15.55 ± 1.14	0.75 ± 0.03
DualGAN, $\sigma = 2$	77.39 ± 7.63	15.54 ± 1.21	0.74 ± 0.04
DualGAN, $\sigma = 5$	77.34 ± 6.65	15.79 ± 1.26	0.75 ± 0.04
DualGAN, $\sigma = 20$	77.16 ± 7.18	15.53 ± 1.27	0.74 ± 0.04
DualGAN with SRGAN (MRI)	71.37 ± 0.29	16.19 ± 0.78	0.76 ± 0.03
DualGAN with SRGAN (CT)	71.99 ± 3.86	16.68 ± 0.92	0.77 ± 0.03
DualGAN with SRGAN (MRI & CT)	65.66 ± 2.30	16.79 ± 0.90	0.78 ± 0.02
DualGAN, VGG, CC	60.83 ± 2.20	17.21 ± 1.00	0.80 ± 0.03
DualGAN, VGG, CC, $\sigma = 1$	71.46 ± 6.15	16.51 ± 1.32	0.77 ± 0.03
DualGAN, VGG, CC, $\sigma = 2$	69.31 ± 6.75	16.29 ± 1.14	0.76 ± 0.04
DualGAN, VGG, CC, $\sigma = 5$	75.67 ± 6.07	16.06 ± 1.20	0.75 ± 0.04
DualGAN, VGG, CC, $\sigma = 20$	70.06 ± 1.17	16.03 ± 0.64	0.76 ± 0.03
DualGAN, VGG, CC, SRGAN (MRI)	63.72 ± 2.39	17.11 ± 0.90	0.78 ± 0.03
DualGAN, VGG, CC, SRGAN (CT)	64.81 ± 2.22	17.26 ± 1.15	0.78 ± 0.02
DualGAN, VGG, CC, SRGAN (MRI & CT)	63.75 ± 1.93	17.09 ± 1.05	0.80 ± 0.02

The comparison of the DualGAN, VGG, CC and models presented in literature can be seen in Table 4. The values were obtained from similar experiments on radiology translation tasks [12, 21, 23]. The proposed in this paper architecture has the lowest PSNR: 17.21 dB. Nevertheless, it outperforms other methods by structure similarity - 0.8 and MAE - 60.83 HU. However, the visual quality of the generated images by DualGAN seem to be worse than the original results of CycleGAN translation [21] likely because our datasets contain fewer images of the same anatomical regions in both MRI and CT domains and samples with non-completely overlapping regions.

Table 4. Comparison of synthesis by DualGAN, VGG, CC with other works.

	DualGAN, VGG, CC	CycleGAN [21]	RF [12]	UNIT [23]	Harmonic [23]
	MRI → CT			Flair → T1	
MAE, HU ↓	60.83 ± 2.20	74.44 ± 1.80	60.87 ± 15.10	-	-
PSNR, dB ↑	17.21 ± 1.00	15.96 ± 0.89	24.63 ± 1.73	25.11	27.22
SSIM ↑	0.80 ± 0.03	0.77 ± 0.03	-	0.76	0.76

5   Conclusion

The DualGAN, VGG, CC model achieved MAE of 60.83 HU, PSNR of 17.21 dB and SSIM of 0.8, which is comparable to scientific literature. Our architecture retains structural information in an image and works with unpaired MRI-CT data. While the DualGAN, VGG and the DualGAN, CC combos are not themselves superior to the DualGAN model, their combination proved to be the best performing architecture. The SRGAN and Unsharp masking, either for pre-processing or for post-processing, did not improve the quality of the generated images. Visual examination by experts confirmed that the perceptual loss term and the coordinate convolutional layer enhanced the appearance of the synthetic images. The translation error was found to depend on the complexity of the head features. The MRI-CT translation approach holds potential to eliminate the need to conduct both imaging procedures and can streamline the workflow of radiotherapy planning.

Acknowledgement. Data used in this publication were generated by the National Cancer Institute Clinical Proteomic Tumor Analysis Consortium (CPTAC).

References

1. Battista, J.J., Rider, W.D., Van Dyk, J.: Computed tomography for radiotherapy planning. Int. J. Radiat. Oncol.* Biol.* Phys. **6**(1), 99–107 (1980)
2. Chen, L., et al.: MRI-based treatment planning for radiotherapy: dosimetric verification for prostate IMRT. Int. J. Radiat. Oncol.* Biol.* Phys. **60**(2), 636–647 (2004)
3. Clark, K., et al.: The cancer imaging archive (TCIA): maintaining and operating a public information repository. J. Digit. Imaging **26**(6), 1045–1057 (2013)
4. Coy, P., Kennelly, G.: The role of curative radiotherapy in the treatment of lung cancer. Cancer **45**(4), 698–702 (1980)

5. (CPTAC), N.C.I.C.P.T.A.C.: Radiology Data from the Clinical Proteomic Tumor Analysis Consortium Glioblastoma Multiforme [CPTAC-GBM] collection [Data set]. The Cancer Imaging Archive (2018). https://doi.org/10.7937/k9/tcia.2018. 3rje41q1

6. Gelband, H., Jha, P., Sankaranarayanan, R., Horton, S.: Disease Control Priorities: Cancer, vol. 3. The World Bank (2015)

7. Hofmann, M., et al.: MRI-based attenuation correction for PET/MRI: a novel approach combining pattern recognition and atlas registration. J. Nucl. Med. **49**(11), 1875–1883 (2008)

8. Johnson, J., Alahi, A., Fei-Fei, L.: Perceptual losses for real-time style transfer and super-resolution. In: Leibe, B., Matas, J., Sebe, N., Welling, M. (eds.) ECCV 2016. LNCS, vol. 9906, pp. 694–711. Springer, Cham (2016). https://doi.org/10. 1007/978-3-319-46475-6_43

9. Kapanen, M., Collan, J., Beule, A., Seppälä, T., Saarilahti, K., Tenhunen, M.: Commissioning of MRI-only based treatment planning procedure for external beam radiotherapy of prostate. Magn. Reson. Med. **70**(1), 127–135 (2013)

10. Karlsson, M., Karlsson, M.G., Nyholm, T., Amies, C., Zackrisson, B.: Dedicated magnetic resonance imaging in the radiotherapy clinic. Int. J. Radiat. Oncol.* Biol.* Phys. **74**(2), 644–651 (2009)

11. Ledig, C., et al.: Photo-realistic single image super-resolution using a generative adversarial network. CoRR abs/1609.04802 (2016)

12. Lei, Y., et al.: MRI-based pseudo CT synthesis using anatomical signature and alternating random forest with iterative refinement model. J. Med. Imaging **5**(4), 043504 (2018)

13. Liu, M., Breuel, T., Kautz, J.: Unsupervised image-to-image translation networks. CoRR abs/1703.00848 (2017). http://arxiv.org/abs/1703.00848

14. Liu, R., et al.: An intriguing failing of convolutional neural networks and the coordconv solution. arXiv preprint arXiv:1807.03247 (2018)

15. Mph, R.L.S., Kimberly, D.: Cancer statistics, 2017. CA Cancer J. Clin. **67**(1), 7–30 (2017)

16. Polesel, A., Ramponi, G., Mathews, V.J.: Image enhancement via adaptive unsharp masking. IEEE Trans. Image Process. **9**(3), 505–510 (2000)

17. Prokopenko, D., Stadelmann, J.V., Schulz, H., Renisch, S., Dylov, D.V.: Synthetic CT generation from MRI using improved DualGAN (2019)

18. Ren, H.: SRGAN: A PyTorch implementation of SRGAN based on CVPR 2017 paper photo-realistic single image super-resolution using a generative adversarial network

19. Vallières, M., et al.: Radiomics strategies for risk assessment of tumour failure in head-and-neck cancer. Sci. Rep. **7**(1), 10117 (2017)

20. Vallières, M., et al.: Data from Head-Neck-PET-CT. The Cancer Imaging Archive (2017). https://doi.org/10.7937/K9/TCIA.2017.8oje5q00

21. Wolterink, J.M., Dinkla, A.M., Savenije, M.H.F., Seevinck, P.R., van den Berg, C.A.T., Isgum, I.: Deep MR to CT synthesis using unpaired data. CoRR abs/1708.01155 (2017). http://arxiv.org/abs/1708.01155

22. Yi, Z., Zhang, H., Tan, P., Gong, M.: DualGAN: unsupervised dual learning for image-to-image translation. CoRR abs/1704.02510 (2017)

23. Zhang, R., Pfister, T., Li, J.: Harmonic unpaired image-to-image translation. In: ICLR (2019)

24. Zhu, J.Y., Park, T., Isola, P., Efros, A.A.: Unpaired image-to-image translation using cycle-consistent adversarial networks. arXiv preprint (2017)

Deriving Lung Perfusion Directly from CT Image Using Deep Convolutional Neural Network: A Preliminary Study

Ge Ren[1], Wai Yin Ho[2], Jing Qin[3], and Jing Cai[1(✉)]

[1] Department of Health Technology and Informatics,
The Hong Kong Polytechnic University, Hung Hom, Hong Kong
jing.cai@polyu.edu.hk
[2] Department of Nuclear Medicine, Queen Mary Hospital,
Pok Fu Lam, Hong Kong
[3] School of Nursing, The Hong Kong Polytechnic University,
Hung Hom, Hong Kong

Abstract. Functional avoidance radiation therapy for lung cancer patients aims to limit dose delivery to highly functional lung. However, the clinical functional imaging suffers from many shortcomings, including the need of exogenous contrasts, longer processing time, etc. In this study, we present a new approach to derive the lung functional images, using a deep convolutional neural network to learn and exploit the underlying functional information in the CT image and generate functional perfusion image. In this study, ^{99m}Tc MAA SPECT/CT scans of 30 lung cancer patients were retrospectively analyzed. The CNN model was trained using randomly selected dataset of 25 patients and tested using the remaining 5 subjects. Our study showed that it is feasible to derive perfusion images from CT image. Using the deep neural network with discrete labels, the main defect regions can be predicted. This technique holds the promise to provide lung function images for image guided functional lung avoidance radiation therapy.

Keywords: Perfusion imaging · Functional avoidance radiation therapy · Deep learning

1 Introduction

Lung cancer is the most common occurring cancer among adults worldwide, with the most common cancer-related death (1.7 million in 2018) [1]. Approximately 85% of lung cancer patients were diagnosed with non-small cell lung cancer (NSCLC), of which 30%–50% were locally advanced (Stage III) NSCLC with median survival of 29 months [2, 3]. The standard treatment for locally advanced NSCLC is concurrent chemoradiotherapy, but the long-term survival is impaired by a high rate of local failure [4]. The clinical practice to achieve local control is dose-escalation above the standard 60 Gy. However, giving more dose to the functional lung would increase the risk of radiation-induced lung injury, which involves radiation pneumonitis in the acute term and pulmonary fibrosis in the long term [5].

© Springer Nature Switzerland AG 2019
D. Nguyen et al. (Eds.): AIRT 2019, LNCS 11850, pp. 102–109, 2019.
https://doi.org/10.1007/978-3-030-32486-5_13

To avoid these side effects, functional avoidance radiation therapy for lung cancer patients was brought out to limit dose delivery to highly functional lung [6]. In this process, images with lung functional information was needed to differentiate function and non-function regions. In clinical practice, the standard test of regional lung function were ventilation and perfusion imaging [7]. Clinical ventilation imaging, such as ^{99m}Tc SPECT [8], ^{68}Ga PET [9], and hyperpolarized ^{3}He gas MRI [10] are generally of low accessibility for the radiation oncology departments, invasive techniques, high cost. Therefore, clinical practice of these three modalities are limited. Deriving ventilation map from 4DCT deformation fields also suffer from large variance from different registration algorithms [11].

Perfusion SPECT/CT imaging has been commonly utilized as a predictor of pulmonary function after surgery [12]. It also has potential for treatment planning in functional lung avoidance radiation therapy. Technetium-99m-labeled macroaggregated albumin (^{99m}Tc MAA) provides a quantitative measure of regional variation in pulmonary perfusion. Besides perfusion SPECT imaging, a more convenient method is to derive the perfusion map from the CT images, which is a routinely utilized for radiation treatment planning. CT-based perfusion imaging does not require exogenous contrast anymore. This method is based on image processing of lung CT images acquired during tidal breathing or breath-hold procedures, and it should be able to transform CT from purely anatomic modality into one that can image and quantify lung perfusion. Since the CT Hounsfield Unit (HU) values is a function of the fractional air/tissue ratio [13], a deep learning model could hold the promise to extract the underlying information of translating the HU values into functional perfusion images. In the field of radiation therapy, deep learning-based convolutional neural network (CNN) has been successfully applied in low-dose CT image correction [14, 15], MR-to-CT image synthesis [16], image segmentation [17, 18], and so on. CNN has found to be able to learn and exploit the underlying features that cannot be extracted by conventional image-processing methods [19]. CNN-based CT perfusion imaging has great promise to improve the toxicity outcomes of lung cancer radiation therapy by enabling perfusion-guided treatment planning that minimizes irradiation of functional lung.

This study aims to explore the feasibility of using deep neural network to derive perfusion-based pulmonary functional images from lung CT images. The proposed method utilized CNN to extract the air/tissue ratio information in the CT images and then used the underlying information to generate functional perfusion images. Our study showed that it is feasible to drive perfusion images from CT image. The performance of CNN with data discretization was superior over the CNN with data reduction by testing on our dataset. Given the performance of the preliminary study and computational efficiency of this method, the proposed deep learning method could hold significant value for future functional avoidance radiation therapy.

2   Materials and Methods

2.1   Patients and Image Acquisition

In this study, ^{99m}Tc MAA SPECT/CT scans of 30 lung cancer patients were retrospectively analyzed. The use of the scan data and waivers of onset were approved by the Queen Mary Hospital (Hong Kong). Patients were immobilized in the supine position with the normal resting breathing. Each scan covered the whole lung volume. The CT images were reconstructed in 512×512 matrix with 0.977×0.977 mm^2 pixel spacing, and 1.25 mm slice spacing. The SPECT images were reconstructed in $128 \times 128 \times 128$ matrix with $4.42 \times 4.42 \times 4.42$ mm^3 voxel size. SPECT images were anatomically registered with the CT images.

2.2   Data Preprocessing

Image Preparation. Initially, SPECT images were resampled at the CT geometry. We built a lung mask to represent the lung parenchyma tissue. This mask included voxels of CT values <-300 HU growing from the lung region, and the trachea was manually excluded from the lung mask. For all cases, the primary lung tumor volume was not included from the lung mask. The lung mask was subsequently applied on the SPECT and CT images to segment the parenchyma volume. The segmented images were further cropped to include only the lung and resized to $128 \times 128 \times 64$ matrix to reduce the consumption of the computation power. For both the SPECT and CT images, a 3D median filter within a cubic region of dimension $6 \times 6 \times 6$ (cube width ~ 18 mm) was applied around each lung voxel for better feature selection.

Data Labelling. To normalize the SPECT values in different patients, all voxels values were divided by the 90th percentile value in the lung. Voxels with value of outlier were set with the threshold values. Our CNN was trained to derive the low function regions from the processed CT images so that the normal regions can be derived. Hence, we first obtained the training datasets consisting of paired input and

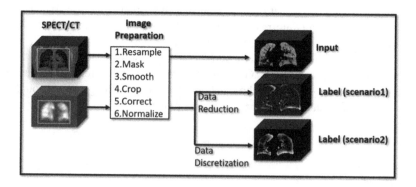

Fig. 1. Diagram of data preprocessing workflow.

output data. Since the purpose of this study was to predict the non-functional lung region.

Then, two labelling approaches were used to compare the performance of the network with different processed data. For the first scenario, voxels with values over 0.5 were excluded from the label map. The rest of the voxels were rescaled from 0 to 1. This method selected only a subset of the most important information from the SPECT images. For the second scenario, continuous values of the SPECT images were converted into 11 intervals with range of [0, 0.1, 0.2, ... 1].

2.3   Neural Network Architecture

We used a 3D U-net [20] based CNN to learn underlying information in the training phase and translate CT images into lung perfusion images in the testing phase. This CNN includes 2 sequential paths (see Fig. 1). The contraction path, which captures the context in CT images, has 5 sequential layers. Each layer consists of a leaky rectified linear unit (leaky ReLU) as an activation function, followed by $3 \times 3 \times 3$ convolution for detecting features, and $2 \times 2 \times 2$ stride convolution for downsampling. The expansion path, which enables precise localization, consists of the leaky ReLU, $3 \times 3 \times 3$ convolution, $1 \times 1 \times 1$ convolution, and $2 \times 2 \times 2$ transpose convolution. The element-wise sum array layer was used before the Sigmoid activation function to sum $3 \times 3 \times 3$ convolution results of the previous layers. The predicted values are in the range of [0, 1]. Symmetric skip connections was used to translate the local details captured in the feature maps from the contraction path into the expansion path. The dropout and early stopping were used to avoid overfitting. This network was implemented using the Pytorch 1.1 framework (Fig. 2).

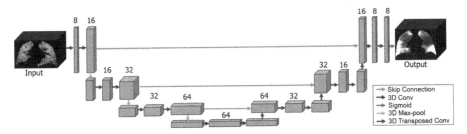

Fig. 2. CNN architecture. The blue indicates the feature map. Blue arrows represent three-dimensional (3D) convolutional layers with 3×3 filter. Red and green arrows indicate 3D max pooling and transposed convolution respectively. Orange arrow indicate sigmoid layer. The numbers on the top of the box indicate the number of channels. (Color figure online)

2.4   Network Training

The network was trained using randomly selected dataset of 25 patients and tested using data from the remaining 5 subjects. Image flip was randomly applied to augment the training datasets during training. The processed CT and SPECT images were used for network training and validation. All the input and output datasets were in 3D volume format. The mean square error was used as the loss function. Each layer was updated using error back-propagation with adaptive moment estimation optimizer (ADAM). The loss function used in this study was binary cross entropy. The learning rate for determining to what extent the newly acquired information overrides the old information was initially 10E−5. The number of epochs was 10000 and each epoch includes 2 iterations. The network was trained on one GTX 2080 TI GPU.

2.5   Evaluation

The generated perfusion images were compared with the perfusion label images from the testing groups. In this study, the correlation coefficient (Spearman's r) metric was used to compare the two images. The Spearman correlation coefficient r was defined using the following equation:

$$r = \frac{\sum_i (I_i - \bar{I})(I_i^* - \bar{I}^*)}{\sqrt{\sum_i (I_i - \bar{I})^2 \sum_i (I_i^* - \bar{I}^*)^2}} \tag{1}$$

where the notation I denotes the generated perfusion obtained using the network. I^* denotes perfusion label. The r values were in the range [−1, 1] and represent the intensity monotonicity of spatially correlated voxels.

3   Results

For each testing case, we calculated the correlation coefficients of scenario 1 and scenario 2. Table 1 shows the correlation values of the prediction and labels. The average correlation value of scenario 1 is 0.53, which is larger than the average of scenario 2. Scenario 1 and scenario 2 have the same deviation. Considering that scenario 2 only predicts the functional lung regions, the correlation values is expected to be larger than those in scenario 1, which predicts the whole lung volume. This suggests the performance of CNN with data discretization is superior over the CNN with data reduction by testing on our data set. The correlations between the label and prediction demonstrated a moderate positive correlation for both scenarios.

Table 1. Correlation values between predicted and label images in 5 testing cases.

Case	1	2	3	4	5	Average ± S.D.
Scenario 1	0.45	0.65	0.32	0.63	0.62	0.53 ± 0.14
Scenario 2	0.18	0.43	0.37	0.51	0.42	0.39 ± 0.14

We also visualized two cases for qualitative analysis using the procedure mentioned in scenario 1. As shown in Figs. 3 and 4, most regions of the defects on the upper lobe of right lung were correctly labelled (red arrows). These images demonstrate good correspondence in the low/high function regions between the label and predicted image. For the data reduction case (Fig. 5), the defects on the lower lobe of right/left lung were not predicted. The result from qualitative analysis is in consistent with the correlation values, suggesting data discretization is superior over the data reduction by testing on our data set.

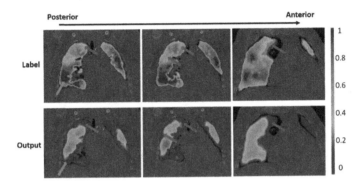

Fig. 3. Comparison of the discrete label and output of case 4 in scenario 1. All images have been normalized using the procedure mentioned in the method section. Red arrows indicate the correctly prediction. Yellow arrows indicate the incorrect prediction. (Color figure online)

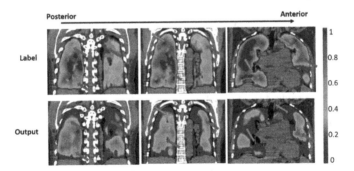

Fig. 4. Comparison of the label and output of case 5 in scenario 1. All images have been normalized using the procedure mentioned in the method section. Red arrows indicate the correctly prediction. Yellow arrows indicate the incorrect prediction. (Color figure online)

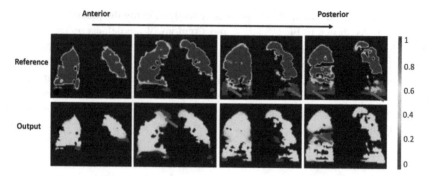

Fig. 5. Comparison of the reduced label and output of case 2 in scenario 2. All images have been normalized using the procedure mentioned in the method section. Red arrows indicate the clinical defect regions. (Color figure online)

4 Summary

Our preliminary study successfully demonstrated the feasibility to derive perfusion images from CT image. Using the deep neural network with discrete label, the main defect regions can be predicted. This technique holds the promise to provide lung functional images for functional lung avoidance radiation therapy.

References

1. Ferlay, J., et al.: Estimating the global cancer incidence and mortality in 2018: GLOBOCAN sources and methods. Int. J. Cancer **144**(8), 1941–1953 (2019)
2. Midha, A., Dearden, S., McCormack, R.: EGFR mutation incidence in non-small-cell lung cancer of adenocarcinoma histology: a systematic review and global map by ethnicity (mutMapII). Am. J. Cancer Res. **5**(9), 2892–2911 (2015)
3. Bradley, J.D., et al.: Standard-dose versus high-dose conformal radiotherapy with concurrent and consolidation carboplatin plus paclitaxel with or without cetuximab for patients with stage IIIA or IIIB non-small-cell lung cancer (RTOG 0617): a randomised, two-by-two factorial phase 3 study. Lancet Oncol. **16**(2), 187–199 (2015)
4. Lee, E., et al.: Functional lung avoidance and response-adaptive escalation (FLARE) RT: Multimodality plan dosimetry of a precision radiation oncology strategy. Med. Phys. **44**(7), 3418–3429 (2017)
5. Madani, I., De Ruyck, K., Goeminne, H., De Neve, W., Thierens, H., Van Meerbeeck, J.: Predicting risk of radiation-induced lung injury. J. Thorac. Oncol. **2**(9), 864–874 (2007)
6. Hoover, D.A., et al.: Functional lung avoidance for individualized radiotherapy (FLAIR): study protocol for a randomized, double-blind clinical trial. BMC Cancer **14**, 934 (2014)
7. Harders, S.W., Balyasnikowa, S., Fischer, B.M.: Functional imaging in lung cancer. Clin. Physiol. Funct. Imaging **34**(5), 340–355 (2014)
8. Suga, K.: Technical and analytical advances in pulmonary ventilation SPECT with xenon-133 gas and Tc-99m-Technegas. Ann. Nucl. Med. **16**(5), 303–310 (2002). (in English)

9. Callahan, J., et al.: High-resolution imaging of pulmonary ventilation and perfusion with 68Ga-VQ respiratory gated (4-D) PET/CT. Eur. J. Nucl. Med. Mol. Imaging **41**(2), 343–349 (2014)
10. Mathew, L., et al.: Hyperpolarized (3)He magnetic resonance imaging: comparison with four-dimensional x-ray computed tomography imaging in lung cancer. Acad. Radiol. **19**(12), 1546–1553 (2012)
11. Kipritidis, J., et al.: The VAMPIRE challenge: a multi-institutional validation study of CT ventilation imaging. Med. Phys. **46**(3), 1198–1217 (2019). (in English)
12. Gefter, W.B., Hatabu, H.: Functional lung imaging: emerging methods to visualize regional pulmonary physiology. Acad. Radiol. **10**(10), 1085–1089 (2003)
13. Kipritidis, J., et al.: Estimating lung ventilation directly from 4D CT Hounsfield unit values. Med. Phys. **43**(1), 33 (2016)
14. Chen, H., et al.: Low-Dose CT with a residual encoder-decoder convolutional neural network. IEEE Trans. Med. Imaging **36**(12), 2524–2535 (2017)
15. Wolterink, J.M., Leiner, T., Viergever, M.A., Isgum, I.: Generative adversarial networks for noise reduction in low-dose CT. IEEE Trans. Med. Imaging **36**(12), 2536–2545 (2017)
16. Jin, C.B., et al.: Deep CT to MR synthesis using paired and unpaired data. Sensors **19**(10), 2361 (2019). (in English)
17. Leung, K., et al.: A deep-learning-based fully automated segmentation approach to delineate tumors in FDG-PET images of patients with lung cancer. J. Nucl. Med. **59**, 323 (2018). (in English)
18. Shin, H.C., et al.: Deep convolutional neural networks for computer-aided detection: CNN architectures, dataset characteristics and transfer learning. IEEE Trans. Med. Imaging **35**(5), 1285–1298 (2016). (in English)
19. Zhong, Y., et al.: Technical note: deriving ventilation imaging from 4DCT by deep convolutional neural network. Med. Phys. **46**(5), 2323–2329 (2019). (in English)
20. Ronneberger, O., Fischer, P., Brox, T.: U-Net: convolutional networks for biomedical image segmentation. In: Navab, N., Hornegger, J., Wells, W.M., Frangi, A.F. (eds.) MICCAI 2015. LNCS, vol. 9351, pp. 234–241. Springer, Cham (2015). https://doi.org/10.1007/978-3-319-24574-4_28

Individualized 3D Dose Distribution Prediction Using Deep Learning

Jianhui Ma[1,2], Ti Bai[2], Dan Nguyen[2], Michael Folkerts[2], Xun Jia[2], Weiguo Lu[2], Linghong Zhou[1(✉)], and Steve Jiang[2(✉)]

[1] Southern Medical University, Guangzhou 510515, Guangdong, China
smart@smu.edu.cn
[2] University of Texas Southwestern Medical Center, Dallas, TX 75390, USA
Steve.Jiang@UTSouthwestern.edu

Abstract. In cancer radiotherapy, inverse treatment planning is a multi-objective optimization problem. There exists a set of plans with various trade-offs on Pareto surface which are referred as Pareto optimal plans. Currently exploring such trade-offs, i.e., physician preference is a trial and error process and often time-consuming. Therefore, it is desirable to predict desired Pareto optimal plans in an efficient way before treatment planning. The predicted plans can be used as references for dosimetrists to rapidly achieve a clinically acceptable plan. Clinically the dose volume histogram (DVH) is a useful tool that can visually indicate the specific dose received by each certain volume percentage which is supposed to describe different trade-offs. Consequently, we have proposed a deep learning method based on patient's anatomy and DVH information to predict the individualized 3D dose distribution. Qualitative measurements have showed analogous dose distributions and DVH curves compared to the true dose distribution. Quantitative measurements have demonstrated that our model can precisely predict the dose distribution with various trade-offs for different patients, with the largest mean and max dose differences between true dose and predicted dose for all critical structures no more than 1.7% of the prescription dose.

Keywords: Deep learning · Treatment planning · Trade-offs · Dose prediction

1 Introduction

Inverse IMRT treatment planning is a multi-objective optimization problem and mathematically can be expressed as the multi-objective weighted least squares function [1]. Various organ weight combinations denoted by trade-offs would lead to a set of plans for a certain patient subject to Pareto surface which are referred as Pareto optimal plans. Currently exploring such trade-offs is a trial and error process and often time-consuming, so it is desirable to predict desired Pareto optimal plans in an efficient way before treatment planning. The predicted plans can be used as references for dosimetrists to rapidly achieve a clinically acceptable plan. Although some approaches have been proposed to work on Pareto optimal plan prediction to guide clinical treatment planning, there are still some deficiencies. The weighted sum methods [2–4] calculate

D. Nguyen et al. (Eds.): AIRT 2019, LNCS 11850, pp. 110–118, 2019.
https://doi.org/10.1007/978-3-030-32486-5_14

the distance between inner and outer approximations of the Pareto surface to minimize the non-negative weighted sum of the objectives, however, they can only work on convex formulations. The epsilon constraint approaches [5–7] firstly apply a single minimization with some constraints to determine a point within a certain region of Pareto surface, and then duplicate the first step using different constraints to seek out a set of points on the Pareto surface. These constraint methods can handle non-convex objective function problem but call for much more time and effort.

In the past few years, deep learning technique has made a great progress and become a research hotspot benefiting from the advancement of graphics cards and theoretical algorithms [8–11]. The fully convolutional network (FCN) [10] adopts the convolutional layers to replace the last several fully-connected layers of traditional CNN for semantic segmentation, and firstly connect deep layers and shallow layers to preserve both global and local features. These innovative ideas make FCN exceed the state-of-the-art in many imaging tasks and many other modified networks are subsequently based on it. In particular, a model known as U-net [11] is proposed for biomedical image segmentation. The U-net consist of two parts: the first part similar to the contracting path of the FCN is designed to extract global features while the second part aims to make a pixel-wise prediction by combining deconvolution output and high-resolution information from the first part, Therefore, the U-net is desired to deal with the challenge of dose distribution prediction. Nguyen et al. [12] firstly explores the feasibility of dose distribution prediction from contours utilizing a modified U-net model. Due to the powerful ability of learning features, they tend to make the model automatically abstract critical features from patient's anatomy without any handcrafted parameters to precisely predict the dose distribution and obtained a remarkable achievement. However, their model just can generate an average conformal dose distribution and cannot account for the physician preference, i.e., different trade-offs. In radiation therapy, the dose volume histogram (DVH) is a useful tool that can visually indicate the specific dose received by each certain volume percentage, the OARs and PTV are denoted by every curve which is supposed to describe different trade-offs for clinical requirements. Therefore, inspired by Dan's groundbreaking work, we'd like to construct a 3D model to focus on the different trade-offs based on patient's anatomy and DVH information. Qualitative and quantitative results demonstrate that our model is promising in individualized dose distribution prediction.

The remainder of this paper is organized as follows. Section 2 firstly introduces the framework of our method and the network architecture. Then, it describes the dataset and the training parameter setting. The performance of dose prediction model is validated in Sect. 3. Section 4 discusses and summarizes the strengths and drawbacks of our model.

2 Methods and Materials

As shown in Fig. 1, the framework of our method consists of two stages: training phase and testing phase. For training dataset (data details seen in Sect. 2.2), each patient possesses multiple Pareto optimal dose distributions and corresponding DVHs which are called feasible DVHs, the DVHs from other patients are considered as infeasible

DVHs. In training phase, the model takes arbitrary (infeasible or feasible) DVHs which are randomly chosen among all training patients and contours as inputs to predict dose distribution. When DVH is feasible, the corresponding dose distribution will be selected as ground truth for supervised learning. If DVH is infeasible, it will be firstly projected to a feasible DVH using a projection method, then the dose distribution corresponding to the feasible DVH is supposed to be true dose distribution as label. The projection method is a l1 norm which is used to measure the distance between infeasible and feasible DVHs to find most similar true dose distribution. In testing phase, any DVHs and contours will be fed into model for dose distribution prediction. The contour image including rectum, bladder, body, and PTV is divided into 4 separate contours which are considered as its own channel, respectively. In this work, we utilize the vector to denote each DVH curve. As we all know, the DVH possesses the properties of dose and corresponding cumulative volume, therefore the critical step is to employ which property of the DVH as the vector value. We have tested both two properties and found that the cumulative volume can represent DVH curve effectively. 4 contour images are encoded with convolution and max-pooling to obtain global feature maps and reduce the feature map size down to the size which can match DVH vector size properly. Meanwhile each DVH curve is converted into a vector whose value is cumulative volume and index represents dose, given that each element in vector indicates a specific dose volume point which can express clinical dose volume constraint, we treat each vector element as a channel. Then DVH vectors and feature maps from contours are concatenated along channel-axis. Finally, the feature fusion maps containing both contour information and DVH information is decoded with deconvolution and convolution to acquire dose distribution. The detailed architecture of encoding and decoding is shown in Fig. 2.

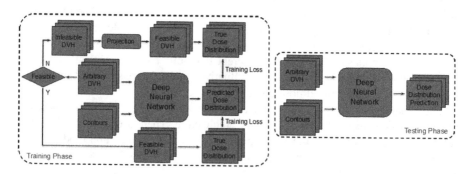

Fig. 1. The workflow of our method

2.1 Architecture

In this study, the modified 3D U-net architecture with encoding (left half) and decoding (right half) is illustrated in Fig. 2. A $3 \times 3 \times 3$ convolutional kernel is applied except for the last two level convolutional layers which use $1 \times 1 \times 1$ kernel instead due to the limitation of the feature map size. Zero padding is applied to keep feature size invariant in the convolution process. 6 max-pooling operations with $2 \times 2 \times 2$ pooling size are employed to reduce the input size from $256 \times 256 \times 64$ to $2 \times 2 \times 1$, and then 1 max-pooling with $2 \times 2 \times 1$ pooling size is utilized to obtain the feature maps with $1 \times 1 \times 1$ size which is equal to the element size in DVH vector. The black dashed rectangle consisting of 4 different color blocks which denote 4 corresponding DVH vectors are concatenated with feature maps from contours along channel-axis. The channel numbers of feature maps from contours and DVHs are equivalent to make them possess same contribution to the final results. Batch normalization [13] is a very efficient way to prevent the gradient from disappearing and accelerate convergence, thus we add batch normalization after the rectified linear unit (ReLU) activated in all layers. Besides, dropout [14] is applied at each convolutional layer to reduce overfitting with randomly deactivating nodes from the network with a certain probability.

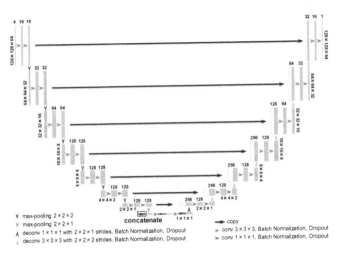

Fig. 2. Modified 3D U-net architecture with two inputs and one output. The green boxes denote multi-channel 3D feature maps while each white box indicates a copied 3D feature map. The number at the top of the box represents channel number for each feature map, and the map size is at the lower left corner of the box. (Color figure online)

2.2 Data and Training Setting

To validate the performance of the model, 97 clinical prostate patients are used here. 10 optimal treatment plans for each patient are generated via a shape-based dose calculation tool which can produce full dose for a given set of fluence maps or calculate a dose matrix for many modalities [15], thus the case amount is 970. Each patient with 4 critical structures comprising rectum, bladder, body, and PTV is subject to a standard

7 beam protocol. The training data contains 77 patients while 20 patients are chosen as testing data. The dimension of contour and dose distribution is $128 \times 128 \times 64$, and each DVH vector contains 32 elements so that the total number of DVH elements is 128 which is also the channel number of contours at the bottom of the network. That is, the input channel of contours is 4 while DVH has 128 input channels. All dose distributions are normalized by PTV mean dose to generate a uniform dataset to benefit training robustness.

As is known to all, the parameters of different networks for various purposes need to be determined manually and empirically. With trial-and-error and fine-tuning, the parameters for our architecture are set as follows. The mean square error (MSE) expressed as Eq. (1) is employed as the loss function to describe the gap between the true dose and the predicted dose.

$$MSE = \frac{1}{N} \sum_{i=1}^{N} \left(D_{true}(i) - D_{pred}(i) \right)^2 \tag{1}$$

where i is the i th voxel in the 3D dose distribution with the total number of voxels N. D_{true} denotes true dose and D_{pred} represents predicted dose.

We adopt the Adam [16] optimization algorithm to minimize the loss function while the initial learning rate is 1×10^{-3}. Considering that big batch size can lead to out of memory error and make the network fall into the local minima, we set the batch size to 3 while it is generally 64 or 128 in the field of image classification and recognition. In this work, we utilized 6 NVIDIA Tesla K80 GPUs to implement our network in Keras library with TensorFlow [17] backend. As shown in Fig. 3, the training loss value can be reduced down to $\sim 1.1618 \times 10^{-4}$ after 300 epochs at the cost of approximately 4 days, more epochs consume much time but achieve very little improvement meanwhile.

3   Results

Figure 3 shows the individualized dose distribution prediction for one patient where each row represents one plan within the same patient. As we can see from the third column, the results predicted a similar dose distribution compared to the true dose, which demonstrated that the model has been capable of characterizing a conformal dose based on patient's anatomy including the shape, size, and location of critical structures. The difference maps between predicted dose and true dose for different plans showed an insignificant gap which meant the model can predict an accurate result. The DVH was generated from the true dose (solid line) and predicted dose distribution (dashed line) where different colors denote different OARs and PTV. Although different DVHs had different trade-offs, the predicted results can still generate a similar trend that covered the curves from true dose well.

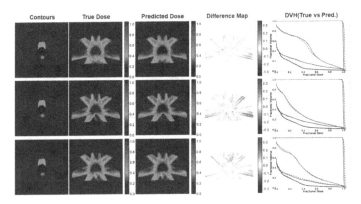

Fig. 3. One example of individualized dose distribution prediction within one patient. From left column to right column: contours, true dose, predicted dose, difference map (true – prediction), and DVH comparing true dose and predicted dose. Each row represents one plan for the same patient.

To clinically evaluate the results, the prescription dose referring to the dose that 95% PTV volumes receive is introduced in the dose difference equation which can be expressed as follows:

$$dose_{difference} = \frac{dose_{true} - dose_{pred}}{dose_{prescription}} \times 100 \tag{2}$$

where $dose_{true}$ denotes the dose of the true dose and $dose_{pred}$ is the predicted dose. The dose difference refers to mean or max dose difference corresponding to $dose_{true}$ and $dose_{pred}$ are denoted by mean dose value or max dose value.

As illustrated in Fig. 4, the boxplot of the mean and max dose differences calculated by the Eq. (2) is plotted for each OAR and PTV across all testing patients including all plans for each patient. The median value denoted by the black line in the box were mildly negative which implied the model slightly over-predicted a dose for the OARs and PTV. To facilitate interpretation, the absolute dose difference statistics (mean value ± standard deviation) were enumerated in Table 1. The max dose differences of body, bladder, rectum, and PTV were 1.22%, 1.59%, 1.13%, and 1.69% of the prescription dose, respectively. The mean dose errors for each critical structure were basically lower than the corresponding max dose errors, ranging from 0.12% for body to 1.58% for PTV. Overall, the absolute dose difference statistics between true dose and predicted dose for all 4 critical structures was no more than 1.7% of the prescription dose.

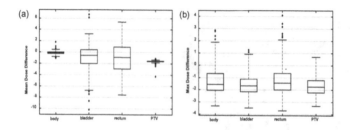

Fig. 4. Boxplot of mean dose difference (a) and max dose difference (b) for all testing patients.

Table 1. Absolute dose difference statistics ($\left|\frac{dose_{true} - dose_{pred}}{dose_{prescription}}\right| \times 100$) for OARs and PTV (mean value $\pm$ standard deviation).

	Mean dose difference	Max dose difference
Body	0.12 ± 0.32	1.22 ± 1.24
Bladder	0.83 ± 2.23	1.59 ± 0.90
Rectum	0.90 ± 2.81	1.13 ± 1.43
PTV	1.58 ± 0.25	1.69 ± 0.78

4   Discussion

In this work, a modified 3D U-net architecture is constructed to predict the individualized dose distribution for different trade-offs. 3D network is suitable for learning essential features of patient's anatomy because the geometry of patient is supposed to be 3D, in contrast, 2D network need to avoid non-coplanar problem by selecting coplanar cases manually. The DVH containing different trade-offs is utilized to guide the network to predict diverse physician preferences for the same patient's anatomy and the contour can lead to a conformal dose, therefore our model integrating them as inputs can yield an individualized conformal dose distribution while the previous work just generates an average dose distribution which cannot handle the different trade-offs. The experimental results have demonstrated that our model can generate a desired result with maintaining the details of dose distribution for different patients as shown in Fig. 3. Dose difference statistics (Fig. 4 and Table 1) show that the model trends to predict an over dose. However, the error is minor where the largest max dose difference is ∼1.69% of the prescription dose and the biggest error in the mean dose is ∼1.58%. Although our model can yield a superior output, there are still some limitations to be solved further. Firstly, patient's anatomy, trade-off, and beam angle are three critical factors for the dose distribution. In this work, the beam angles of the dataset are fixed because our current model cannot account for diverse beam angles, which restricts its scope of application. This is another significant project needs to be solved. Secondly, we just used 10 plans within the same patient to train the model. In other words, our model just has learned a limited range of trade-offs which implies that the model may not predict a satisfied result when the trade-off exceeds the range using in the training phase. Naturally, a method of dealing with this shortcoming is to train the model using more number of treatment plans in order to cover an almost infinite range to yield any trade-off accurately. However, it would spend much more computational time which may be impractical. Furthermore, the clinical region of interest (ROI) actually calls for a limited set of candidates where 10 optimal plans with different trade-offs are enough for physicians.

5   Conclusion

We have proposed a deep learning method based on a modified 3D U-net with patient's anatomy and different trade-offs for treatment planning as inputs to predict an individualized dose distribution. Qualitative measurements have showed analogous dose washes and DVH curves compared to the true dose distribution. Quantitative measurements have demonstrated our model can precisely predict the dose distribution with various trade-offs for different patients, with the largest mean and max dose errors between true dose and predicted dose for the OARs and PTV no more than 1.7% of the prescription dose. In summary, our proposed method has great potential to possess the capability of capturing different trade-offs and patient's anatomy and can provide a guidance for the automatic individualized optimal treatment planning.

References

1. Craft, D.: Multi-criteria optimization methods in radiation therapy planning: a review of technologies and directions. arXiv preprint arXiv:1305.1546 (2013)
2. Rennen, G., van Dam, E.R., den Hertog, D.: Enhancement of sandwich algorithms for approximating higher-dimensional convex Pareto sets. INFORMS J. Comput. 23, 493–517 (2011)
3. Bokrantz, R., Forsgren, A.: An algorithm for approximating convex Pareto surfaces based on dual techniques. INFORMS J. Comput. 25, 377–393 (2013)
4. Bokrantz, R.: Distributed approximation of Pareto surfaces in multicriteria radiation therapy treatment planning. Phys. Med. Biol. 58, 3501 (2013)
5. Miettinen, K.: Nonlinear Multiobjective Optimization, vol. 12. Springer, Heidelberg (2012)
6. Messac, A., Ismail-Yahaya, A., Mattson, C.A.: The normalized normal constraint method for generating the Pareto frontier. Struct. multidisciplinary Optim. 25, 86–98 (2003)
7. Chen, W., Craft, D., Madden, T.M., Zhang, K., Kooy, H.M., Herman, G.T.: A fast optimization algorithm for multicriteria intensity modulated proton therapy planning. Med. Phys. 37, 4938–4945 (2010)
8. LeCun, Y., Boser, B., Denker, J.S., Henderson, D., Howard, R.E., Hubbard, W., et al.: Backpropagation applied to handwritten zip code recognition. Neural Comput. 1, 541–551 (1989)
9. Krizhevsky, A., Sutskever, I., Hinton, G.E.: ImageNet classification with deep convolutional neural networks. In: Advances in Neural Information Processing Systems, pp. 1097–1105 (2012)

10. Long, J., Shelhamer, E., Darrell, T.: Fully convolutional networks for semantic segmentation. In: Proceedings of the IEEE Conference on Computer Vision and Pattern Recognition, pp. 3431–3440 (2015)
11. Ronneberger, O., Fischer, P., Brox, T.: U-Net: convolutional networks for biomedical image segmentation. In: Navab, N., Hornegger, J., Wells, W.M., Frangi, A.F. (eds.) MICCAI 2015. LNCS, vol. 9351, pp. 234–241. Springer, Cham (2015). https://doi.org/10.1007/978-3-319-24574-4_28
12. Nguyen, D., Long, T., Jia, X., Lu, W., Gu, X., Iqbal, Z., et al.: Dose prediction with U-Net: a feasibility study for predicting dose distributions from contours using deep learning on prostate IMRT patients. arXiv preprint arXiv:1709.09233 (2017)
13. Ioffe, S., Szegedy, C.: Batch normalization: accelerating deep network training by reducing internal covariate shift. arXiv preprint arXiv:1502.03167 (2015)
14. Srivastava, N., Hinton, G., Krizhevsky, A., Sutskever, I., Salakhutdinov, R.: Dropout: a simple way to prevent neural networks from overfitting. J. Mach. Learn. Res. **15**, 1929–1958 (2014)
15. Folkerts, M., Long, T., Radke, R., Tian, Z., Jia, X., Chen, M., et al.: WE-AB-207B-07: dose cloud: generating "Big Data" for radiation therapy treatment plan optimization research. Med. Phys. **43**, 3805 (2016)
16. Kingma, D.P., Ba, J.: Adam: a method for stochastic optimization. arXiv preprint arXiv: 1412.6980 (2014)
17. Abadi, M., Agarwal, A., Barham, P., Brevdo, E., Chen, Z., Citro, C., et al.: TensorFlow: large-scale machine learning on heterogeneous distributed systems. arXiv preprint arXiv: 1603.04467 (2016)

Deep Generative Model-Driven Multimodal Prostate Segmentation in Radiotherapy

Kibrom Berihu Girum[1(✉)], Gilles Créhange[1,2], Raabid Hussain[1],
Paul Michael Walker[1,3], and Alain Lalande[1,3]

[1] ImViA, Université de Bourgogne Franche-Comté, Dijon, France
`kibrom-berihu_girum@etu.u-bourgogne.fr`
[2] Department of Radiation Oncology, CGFL, Dijon, France
[3] Depratment of Medical Imaging, University Hospital of Dijon, Dijon, France

Abstract. Deep learning has shown unprecedented success in a variety of applications, such as computer vision and medical image analysis. However, there is still potential to improve segmentation in multimodal images by embedding prior knowledge via learning-based shape modeling and registration to learn the modality invariant anatomical structure of organs. For example, in radiotherapy automatic prostate segmentation is essential in prostate cancer diagnosis, therapy, and post-therapy assessment from T2-weighted MR or CT images. In this paper, we present a fully automatic deep generative model-driven multimodal prostate segmentation method using convolutional neural network (DGMNet). The novelty of our method comes with its embedded generative neural network for learning-based shape modeling and its ability to adapt for different imaging modalities via learning-based registration. The proposed method includes a multi-task learning framework that combines a convolutional feature extraction and an embedded regression and classification based shape modeling. This enables the network to predict the deformable shape of an organ. We show that generative neural network-based shape modeling trained on a reliable contrast imaging modality (such as MRI) can be directly applied to low contrast imaging modality (such as CT) to achieve accurate prostate segmentation. The method was evaluated on MRI and CT datasets acquired from different clinical centers with large variations in contrast and scanning protocols. Experimental results reveal that our method can be used to automatically and accurately segment the prostate gland in different imaging modalities.

Keywords: Prostate segmentation · Convolutional neural network · Transfer learning · Deep learning · CT · MRI

1 Introduction

Automatic segmentation of anatomical structures in medical images has various medical applications. For example, in radiotherapy prostate segmentation is

© Springer Nature Switzerland AG 2019
D. Nguyen et al. (Eds.): AIRT 2019, LNCS 11850, pp. 119–127, 2019.
https://doi.org/10.1007/978-3-030-32486-5_15

essential in the diagnosis, therapy, and post-therapy analysis of prostate cancer. It is critical in selecting patients for a specific treatment, to guide source delivery and in computing dose distribution [1,2]. T2-weighted MRI is the modality of choice for prostate segmentation. However, CT and US are also routinely used because: (1) CT image is used to calculate the dose distribution due to its characteristics of relating the density of tissues with the voxel intensity, and (2) US imaging is suitable for real-time image guided radiotherapy. Despite the need for accurate segmentation of the prostate in radiotherapy, manual segmentation is subjective to inter and intra-observer variabilities, time-consuming, and depends on the experience of the physician. Automatic and reliable segmentation of the prostate on these images is thus an important but difficult task due to the inhomogeneous and inconsistent contrast of prostate boundary and large shape variations. This is particularly complicated on CT images because of the inherent low-contrast imaging characteristics of CT for soft tissues (such as prostate boundary) as can be seen from Fig. 1(b).

Recently, organ boundary detection through modeling and incorporating the organ shape as prior information has been successfully used for automatic and reliable anatomical structure segmentation (such as prostate [1], brain [3], and heart [4]). The prior prostate shape has been modeled using principal component analysis from labeled prostate CT scans. The modeled shape was then used to guide the segmentation of prostate gland on CT images [1]. A deep learning approach followed by a multi-atlas based feature extraction has also been proposed [5]. Distinctive curve guided fully convolutional neural network has also been employed for the pelvic organ segmentation on CT images [6]. Kazemifar et al. [7] used convolutional networks (U-net architecture [8]) to segment both the prostate and organs at risk in male pelvic CT images. Guo et al. [9] have also used deep features and sparse patch matching approach to segment the prostate on MR images. Although atlas and shape-prior based methods demonstrated promising performance, they might not be generic. This lack of generalization ability is due to the possibility of statistical shape or atlas of an organ being different for a new patient. It then requires a robust modeling and registration algorithm. However, robust feature extraction is still a challenging task to obtain an optimal shape model. Indeed in medical images, image contrast, organ shape, acquisition protocol and deformable characteristics of an organ can vary widely.

Deep convolutional neural networks (CNN) have shown promising performances in various medical applications [10]. For example, U-net architecture has been often used for medical image segmentations [8]. Adversarial neural network has also been proven to improve medical image segmentation (e.g. for liver [11]). Thus, our hypothesis is that by combining CNN-based feature extraction and learning-based anatomical structure modeling (through generative neural network) from reliable contrast images (such as T2-weighted MRI for soft tissues), we can predict accurately an organ boundary in low-contrast imaging modalities (e.g. prostate segmentation on CT).

In this paper, we present a new deep generative model-driven anatomical structure segmentation (named DGMNet), specifically designed for multimodal

(CT and MR) prostate segmentation. The proposed method employs a convolutional feature extraction with an embedded generative CNN [8,12]. The generative CNN is designed for learning-based modeling of prior organ shape from MRI and applied to low-contrast CT images. It also involves a learning-based registration with a given raw input image. Experimental results on MRI and CT datasets reveal that our method can fully automatically segment the prostate robustly and accurately regardless of the difference in contrast, size, and imaging modality.

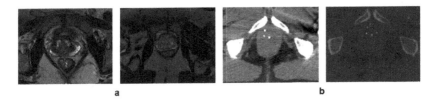

a   b

Fig. 1. Prostate image examples showing image contrast variations in: (a) T2-weighted MRI, and (b) CT images with seeds from low-dose-rate brachytherapy.

2   Methodology

We aim at detecting the boundary of the prostate volume in a given 3D raw input image I of size $W \times H \times C$. Here W, H, and C are width, height and depth of the image, respectively. We use a deep CNN which outputs a label map of size $W \times H \times C$ whose voxels $v = (x, y, z)$ contain a label 1 for prostate volume and 0 otherwise. This is done by combining a predicted label mask from a decoder and a predicted shape from an embedded shape-model generator (see Fig. 2(a)).

2.1   Network Architecture

The network architecture is illustrated in Fig. 2. It consists of feature extraction, generative shape modeling, and feature map upsampling. The feature extraction (encoder) resides on a convolutional neural network [12]. It consists of a repeated application of 3×3 convolution, Rectified Linear Unit (ReLU) activation, batch normalization, followed by squeeze-and-excitation network (SE-Net) [12](see Fig. 2(b)), and a 2×2 max pooling operation with stride 2 for downsampling. From the extracted feature maps, two paths named as model and decoder path are applied. We also used dropout regularization at the bottleneck layer to have a better generalization by reducing over-fitting during the training. The decoder path is composed of a 2×2 up-convolution and concatenation layer, followed by the same block as the encoder (Fig. 2(b)). Generative path (i.e. Model in Fig. 2(a)) is composed of average max pooling followed by fully connected

layers (FC). The output of these FC layers (corresponding to surface boundary coordinates) are feed to the generative model where it generates the shape
of a given organ (in our case, prostate gland). It consists of a projection and
a reshape block followed by repeated Leaky ReLU activation (except the last
activation which was sigmoid), batch normalization, and up-convolution (similar to the one proposed in [13]). The model-generator and decoder outputs are
merged using addition and further a convolutional block is applied. The output
layer is a 1×1 convolutional layer with sigmoid activation function. It is worthy
to mention here that the proposed network involves only 1.5 million trainable
parameters while the U-net architecture has 31.024 million [8].

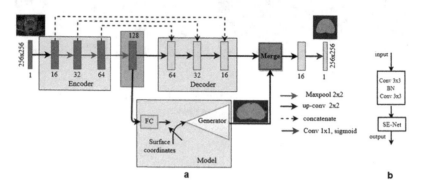

Fig. 2. Proposed architecture: (a) The overall framework (DGMNet), and (b) the
schema of a single block in the encoder and decoder.

Generator: We formulate the model generator to predict the prostate volume
given a few sampled prostate surface boundary coordinates, $I^u = (x^u, y^u, z^u)$. To
this end, the voxel depth (z, for a given slice u) is taken as classification task (0
or 1) and the remaining (x and y) as regression task. Given the surface boundary
coordinates, $I^u = (x^u, y^u, z^u)$, it is trained to predict a labeled model $W \times H \times C$,
in which the prostate volume is 1 and 0 otherwise, i.e. $G(I^u) \mapsto W \times H \times C$. We
automatically extracted four surface boundary landmark coordinates (left, right,
top, and bottom) per-slice from the given labeled ground truth (from MRI) and
repeated over the whole volume of the prostate (I^u).

2.2 Loss Function

To train the proposed network, we define a multi-task loss function as a combined
weighted sum loss:

$$L_{total} = L_{mask} + \lambda L_{clsLnd} , \tag{1}$$

in which the segmentation (final mask) loss, L_{mask}, is calculated as a combination of Dice and cross entropy loss ($L_{mask} = L_{dice} + L_{CE}$).

Given ground truth surface voxel coordinates $I^u = (x^u, y^u, z^u)$, where $z^u = 1$, and predicted values, $I^v = (x^v, y^v, z^v = p)$, the joint classification and regression loss can be calculated as:

$$L_{clsLnd}(I^u, I^v) = L_{cls}(p, z^u) + [z^u = 1]L_{lnd}(t^u, t^v), \qquad (2)$$

in which the classification loss, $L_{cls}(p, z^u)$, is the cross entropy loss. The likelihood of a given raw input image slice (I^u), being part of the organ is p. The ground-truth label, z^u, is 1 if the image slice consists of the prostate, and is 0 otherwise. The second loss, $L_{lnd}(I^u, I^v)$, is thus defined over the surface landmarks where the ground truth is 1 and 0 otherwise. For positive ground truth (i.e. $z^u = 1$), we use smooth $L1$ loss between corresponding voxels, which is considered as robust loss to outliers [14], as:

$$L_{lnd}(t^u, t^v) = \sum_{i \in \{x, y, z=1\}} smooth_{L1}(t_i^u - t_i^v), \qquad (3)$$

in which

$$smooth_{L1}(\Delta t) = \begin{cases} 0.5(\Delta t)^2 & \text{if } |\Delta t| < 1 \\ |\Delta t| - 0.5 & \text{otherwise}, \end{cases} \qquad (4)$$

where $t^u = (x^u, y^u)$ and $t^v = (x^v, y^v)$ are the ground truth and predicted surface boundary coordinates, respectively, for given $z^u = 1$. The hyper-parameter λ controls the losses contributed from the segmentation and surface boundary coordinates.

3   Experimental Setup and Results

3.1   Datasets

The proposed method was trained and evaluated on T2-weighted MRI and CT prostate images with vast variability in organ size, shape, scanning protocol, and from multiple clinical centers. Firstly, it was trained and evaluated on 60 T2-weighted MR exams. These datasets were acquired with an in-plane resolution ranging from 0.312×0.312 mm^2 to 0.676×0.676 mm^2 with a slice thickness between 1.250 mm and 2.722 mm. Similarly, we also trained and evaluated on 40 CT patient datasets (who underwent permanent prostate brachytherapy with ^{125}I for localized prostate cancer treatment). These CT exams were acquired from two clinical centers. The in-plane resolution of these CT data varies from 0.4×0.4 mm^2 to 0.58×0.58 mm^2 with a slice thickness between 1.5 mm and 2.5 mm (helical mode, 120 kVp, 172 mm FOV, and 440 mAs/slice). We looked for conversions of the datasets into the same voxel size of $0.5 \times 0.5 \times 1.25$ mm^3 and $0.7 \times 0.7 \times 1.25$ mm^3 for CT and MRI respectively. The prostate was manually delineated by experienced radiologists.

Pre-processing: The input images (MR and CT) were pre-processed by zero-centering the intensity values and normalizing them by the standard deviation of all images before feeding to the network. All images were also center cropped and resized to have an image resolution of 256×256.

Training and Testing Details: We trained the system by minimizing the loss L_{total} (Eq. 1). The proposed system is trained as follows: (1) Firstly, we train the generative model with the inputs from a few sampled surface boundary landmarks of the prostate volume, specifically from only T2-weighted MRI labels. We used a binary cross entropy loss for training. We conducted five-fold cross validation experiment. (2) Secondly, the whole system is trained except the generator in which it only predicts the model shape given the predicted surface coordinate values from FC network. We use a batch size of 10 images for both MRI and CT. It is important to mention here that we feed the network with 2D instead of 3D as we have small datasets. Then, predicted image labels are stacked to create a 3D volume. The model is trained using Adam optimizer with a learning rate of 0.001. The whole ensembled architecture (except the generator) was trained from scratch considering 10 patients (25% of the datasets which were selected randomly) for validation.

Ablation Study: We conducted ablation experiments (Table 1) to investigate the effect of individual components in the proposed network. All ablation experiments were done on CT images under similar settings: (1) Unet architecture; (2) ResUnet (residual-based Unet); (3) SE-ResUnet (residual block with squeeze-and-excitation network based Unet [12]); (4) SE-Unet (the proposed method without the generator and the FC network (Fig. 2(b))).

Evaluation Metrics: All experiments were evaluated using Dice Similarity Coefficient (DSC), Sensitivity (Sen), positive predicted value (PPV), and average surface distance (ASD) (in mm) [15].

3.2   Experimental Results

The generator was trained using a five-fold cross validation method using T2-weighted MRI. It was then kept as a shape predictor by freezing its weights during training of the proposed method. As this is an intermediate output of the method, it can be considered as a region proposal (or as instantaneous shape generator) to be further refined by merging with the encoder-decoder output. Indeed, the model-generator can learn from good contrast images (MRI) and used directly (transfer without fine tuning by freezing) for low contrast images (CT), while the encoder-decoder extracts additional features. As one can see from the qualitative prostate segmentation results in Fig. 3, the proposed method can segment accurately the prostate on both T2-weighted MR and CT images.

In almost all evaluation metrics (with and without the generator, Table 1), the proposed method with the shape model generator outperforms the state of

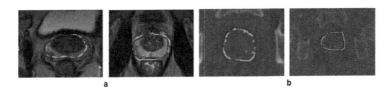

Fig. 3. Qualitative evaluation of prostate segmentation on 2D: (a) T2-weighted MRI, and (b) CT images with seeds from low-dose-rate brachytherapy. The ground truth labels are shown in red and segmentation results in green. (Color figure online)

the art methods. Since the implanted radioactive seeds were not uniformly placed over the volume of the prostate gland, it was observed to influence the segmentation quality (particularly the state of the art methods). However, they might perform better on CT images without the implanted radioactive seeds. Combining CNN-based extracted features with prior shape knowledge of the organ can improve time, reproducibility, and accuracy in fully automatic segmentation of the prostate in radiotherapy.

Table 1. Quantitative segmentation results. Values are expressed as mean ± std.

Data	Method	DSC	Sen	ASD	PPV
CT	Unet	0.83 ± 0.04	0.76 ± 0.08	0.16 ± 0.08	0.93 ± 0.03
	ResUnet	0.82 ± 0.03	0.73 ± 0.03	0.16 ± 0.10	0.93 ± 0.03
	SE-ResUnet	0.84 ± 0.03	0.88 ± 0.05	0.84 ± 0.53	0.82 ± 0.06
	SE-Unet	0.85 ± 0.03	0.78 ± 0.07	0.17 ± 0.15	0.93 ± 0.04
	DGMNet	0.89 ± 0.02	0.92 ± 0.03	0.28 ± 0.09	0.87 ± 0.03
MRI	**DGMNet**	0.93 ± 0.12	0.92 ± 0.15	0.11 ± 0.22	0.96 ± 0.07

4   Conclusion

In this paper we proposed DGMNet, a new CNN approach for feature-model learning based anatomical structure segmentation. It is an encoder-decoder architecture and an embedded deep generative neural network based model-generator that enables training on limited data. The model-generator is used for embedding prior shape knowledge via learning based shape modeling and registration from high contrast images (such as MRI) and directly applied (by freezing) to low contrast images (such as CT). Further, we demonstrated that combining shape-model with a CNN-based feature extraction improves segmentation accuracy. We extensively evaluated models trained with and without prior shape generator on CT images with different metrics to verify the effect of the embedded shape generator. Experimental results, on MR and CT datasets, reveal that this method can be used to fully-automatically segment prostate gland in different imaging modalities. In the future, we plan on generalizing the proposed method to other modalities such as US images (for intra-operative radiotherapy) as well as to other organs (such as rectum, brain, and heart). In the case of US images, we shall propose to train the model-generator from MRI with an endorectal coil to consider the deformation characteristics of the prostate gland from the coil.

References

1. Martnez, F., Romero, E., Dran, G., Simon, A., Haigron, P., De Crevoisier, R., et al.: Segmentation of pelvic structures for planning CT using a geometrical shape model tuned by a multi-scale edge detector. Phys. Med. Biol. **59**(6), 1471 (2014). https://doi.org/10.1088/0031-9155/59/6/1471
2. Girum, K.B., Lalande, A., Quivrin, M., Bessires, I., Pierrat, N., Martin, E., et al.: Inferring postimplant dose distribution of salvage permanent prostate implant (PPI) after primary PPI on CT images. Brachytherapy **17**(6), 866–873 (2018). https://doi.org/10.1016/j.brachy.2018.07.017
3. Ilunga-Mbuyamba, E., Avina-Cervantes, J.G., Lindner, D., Arlt, F., Ituna-Yudonago, J.F., et al.: Patient-specific model-based segmentation of brain tumors in 3D intraoperative ultrasound images. Int. J. Comput. Assist. Radiol. Surg. **13**(3), 331–342 (2018). https://doi.org/10.1007/s11548-018-1703-0
4. Zotti, C., Luo, Z., Lalande, A., Jodoin, P.M.: Convolutional neural network with shape prior applied to cardiac MRI segmentation. IEEE J. Biomed. Health Inform. **23**(3), 1119–1128 (2018). https://doi.org/10.1109/JBHI.2018.2865450
5. Ma, L., Guo, R., Zhang, G., Tade, F., Schuster, D.M., Nieh, P. et al.: Automatic segmentation of the prostate on CT images using deep learning and multi-atlas fusion. In: Medical Imaging 2017: Image Processing, p. 1013320. SPIE (2017). https://doi.org/10.1117/12.2255755
6. He, K., Cao, X., Shi, Y., Nie, D., Gao, Y., Shen, D.: Pelvic organ segmentation using distinctive curve guided fully convolutional networks. IEEE Trans. Med. Imaging **38**(2), 585–595 (2019). https://doi.org/10.1109/TMI.2018.2867837
7. Kazemifar, S., Balagopal, A., Nguyen, D., McGuire, S., Hannan, R., Jiang, S.M., et al.: Segmentation of the prostate and organs at risk in male pelvic CT images using deep learning. Biomed. Phys. Eng. Express **4**(5), 055003 (2018). https://doi.org/10.1088/2057-1976/aad100
8. Ronneberger, O., Fischer, P., Brox, T.: U-Net: convolutional networks for biomedical image segmentation. In: Navab, N., Hornegger, J., Wells, W.M., Frangi, A.F. (eds.) MICCAI 2015. LNCS, vol. 9351, pp. 234–241. Springer, Cham (2015). https://doi.org/10.1007/978-3-319-24574-4_28
9. Guo, Y., Gao, Y., Shen, D.: Deformable MR prostate segmentation via deep feature learning and sparse patch matching. IEEE Trans. Med. Imaging **35**(4), 1077–1089 (2016). https://doi.org/10.1109/TMI.2015.2508280
10. Litjens, G., Kooi, T., Bejnordi, B.E., Setio, A.A.A., Ciompi, F., Ghafoorian, M., et al.: A survey on deep learning in medical image analysis. Med. Image Anal. **42**, 60–88 (2017). https://doi.org/10.1016/j.media.2017.07.005
11. Yang, D., et al.: Automatic liver segmentation using an adversarial image-to-image network. In: Descoteaux, M., Maier-Hein, L., Franz, A., Jannin, P., Collins, D.L., Duchesne, S. (eds.) MICCAI 2017. LNCS, vol. 10435, pp. 507–515. Springer, Cham (2017). https://doi.org/10.1007/978-3-319-66179-7_58

12. Hu, J., Shen, L., Sun, G.: Squeeze-and-excitation networks. In: CVPR, pp. 7132–7141 (2018). https://doi.org/10.1109/CVPR.2018.00745
13. Radford, A., Metz, L., Chintala, S.: Unsupervised representation learning with deep convolutional generative adversarial networks. In: ICLR (2016)
14. He, K., Gkioxari, G., Dollr, P., Girshick, R.: Mask R-CNN. In: ICCV, pp. 2961–2969 (2017). https://doi.org/10.1109/TPAMI.2018.2844175
15. Litjens, G., Toth, R., van de Ven, W., Hoeks, C., Kerkstra, S., van Ginneken, B., et al.: Evaluation of prostate segmentation algorithms for MRI: the PROMISE12 challenge. Med. Image Anal. **18**(2), 359–373 (2014). https://doi.org/10.1016/j.media.2013.12.002

Dose Distribution Prediction for Optimal Treamtment of Modern External Beam Radiation Therapy for Nasopharyngeal Carcinoma

Bilel Daoud[1($\boxtimes$)], Ken'ichi Morooka[1], Shoko Miyauchi[1], Ryo Kurazume[1], Wafa Mnejja[2], Leila Farhat[2], and Jamel Daoud[2]

[1] Graduate School of Information Science and Electrical Engineering, Kyushu University, Fukuoka, Japan
daoud@irvs.ait.kyushu-u.ac.jp
[2] Radiotherapy Department of Habib Bourguiba Hospital, Sfax, Tunisia

Abstract. In Intensity-modulated radiation therapy, the planning of the optimal dose distribution for a patient is a complex and time-consuming process. This paper proposes a new automatic method for predicting of dose distribution of Nasopharyngeal carcinoma (NPC) from contoured computer tomography (CT) images. The proposed method consists of two phases: (1) predicting the 2D optimal dose images of each beam from contoured CT images of a patient by convolutional deep neural network model, called OTNet, and (2) integrating the optimal dose images of all the beams to predict the dose distribution for the patient. From the experiments using CT images of 80 NPC patients, our proposed method achieves a good performance for predicting dose distribution compared with conventional predicted dose distribution methods.

Keywords: Convolutional neural network · Dose distribution prediction · Nasopharyngeal carcinoma · Intensity-modulated radiation therapy

1 Introduction

Intensity-modulated radiation therapy (IMRT) has been a common method for an external beam radiation treatment for cancers. In IMRT, radiation oncologists can control the intensity of the radiation beam according to the size, shape and location of a target tumor. Owing to this, IMRT enables to achieve adaptive radiotherapy, that is, IMRT destroys tumors with complex shapes by delivering more focused radiation to the tumor or specific areas within the tumor. At the same time, IMRT avoids the exposure of healthy tissues by reducing the radiation dose to the healthy tissues. Therefore, IMRT is recommended for over 50% of all cancers such as nasopharyngeal carcinoma (NPC) to eradicate cancer cells [1].

In IMRT, a patient is irradiated by beams of high energy X-rays (4-20 MV) or electrons (4-25 MeV) from multiple directions. Since the beam damages both

© Springer Nature Switzerland AG 2019
D. Nguyen et al. (Eds.): AIRT 2019, LNCS 11850, pp. 128–136, 2019.
https://doi.org/10.1007/978-3-030-32486-5_16

healthy and cancerous tissue, to minimize the effect of damaging healthy tissue, the prescribed dose of radiation (70 Gy) is usually delivered to a target tumor for 35 days with 2 Gy per day.

Before starting the treatment, radiation oncologists plan a IMRT treatment by using treatment planning systems. Using computed tomography (CT) images of the patient, a set of dose objectives for the tumor and organs at risk (OARs) [2], the treatment planning systems determine a treatment plan including the optimal parameters of each beam and the delivered dose from each aperture. As mentioned above, the optimal IMRT treatment is to deliver more focused radiation to the tumor while reducing the radiation dose to the healthy tissues in order to eradicate all cancer cells without any complications. However, since the current planning systems don't always provide the optimal treatment for a patient, radiation oncologists need to modify the treatment plan repeatedly to obtain a desired dose distribution. This modification process is time-consuming, from several hours to a week. Moreover, the quality of the determined treatment plan highly depends on the knowledges and experiences of the radiation oncologists [3].

Recent researches have been developing optimal IMRT planing techniques [4,5]. Among them, objective-based planning (OBP) [4] uses pre-set objectives of dose to achieve desirable IMRT treatment. As another IMRT planning method, knowledge-based planning (KBP) [5] predicts the dose distribution of a new patient by using a set of previous plans of treated patients. However, these methods require radiation oncologists much effort and time to determine the suitable handcrafted features such as spatial information of OARs and tumors, number of beams and distance to the tumor to obtain a good dose distribution.

Here, deep learning methods using convolutional neural networks (CNNs) have achieved successes in radiotherapy such as automatic segmentation [6] and toxicity prediction of radiotherapy plan [7]. Inspired by this success, CNN is applied to predict radiotherapy plans [8,9]. Mahmood et al. [8] introduced a generative adversarial network (GAN) model to construct the U-net-based generator which predicts the dose distributions from 2D contours of tumor and OARs in CT images. Chen et al. [9] constructed dose distribution prediction system for NPC using ResNet101 whose inputs are CT images with tumors and OARs regions. Although the radiation beam geometry influences on the dose distribution, the two methods [8,9] don't consider the radiation beam geometry. Therefore, the methods in [8,9] strongly depend on the quality of the dose distribution images used in the system construction.

In this paper, we propose a new system for predicting the dose distribution from contoured CT images, called contoured CT images, that contains the countours and regions of tumors and OARs. The proposed system consists of two main processes. Firstly, for each beam, the proposed system estimates a 2D dose image of the beam which shows the dose distribution delivered from the beam orientation. Next, using the dose images of all the beams, the system predicts the dose distribution for a patient by integrating all the dose images. As a result, a 3D dose distribution image is created after the prediction of 2D dose distribution images from CT images of a patient. Through the two processes, the

Table 1. Detailed information of contoured regions and its labels.

Contours	Dose constraint	Label	Contours	Dose constraint	Label
L/R temporomandibular joint (TMJ)	$D_{max} \leq 55$ Gy	1/2	L/R parotid gland	$D_{50} < 26$ Gy	12/13
Optic chiasma	$D_{max} \leq 54$ Gy	3	Brainstem	$D_{1cc} < 54$ Gy	14
L/R Lens	$D_{max} \leq 7$ Gy	4/5	Spinal cord	$D_{1cc} \leq 40$ Gy	15
Larynx	$D_{max} \leq 66$ Gy	6	PTV (70 Gy)	$D_{95\%} \geq 66.5$ Gy	16
Temporal lobe	$D_{2\%} < 60$ Gy	7	GTV (70 Gy)	$D_{98\%} \geq 70$ Gy	17
L/R Mandible	$D_{max} \leq 65$ Gy	8/9	CTV (70 Gy)	$D_{95\%} \geq 70$ Gy	18
L/R optic nerve	$D_{max} \leq 55$ Gy	10/11			

L/R: Left/Right; D_{max}: maximum dose; D_{50}: 50% of the dose, $D_{2\%}$, $D_{95\%}$, $D_{98\%}$: 2%, 95%, 98% of the dose, respectively; D_{1cc}: 1 cubic centimeter of the dose.

proposed method predicts the dose distribution for the patient considering the radiation beam geometry. Because of this advantage, the proposed method can improve the dose prediction accuracy compared with the previous works that don't consider the beam geometry.

2   Methods

2.1   Materials

The dataset used in our method consists of the data of 80 NPC patients diagnosed at Radiotherapy department of Habib Bourguiba Hospital of Sfax-Tunisia. The data of each patient include two components: (1) axial section CT images with 256×256 [pixels] trimmed from 512×512 [pixels] and (2) real dose distribution images for the patient. From each CT image, two radiation oncologists manually extract the regions of the gross tumor volume of the NPC (GTV), clinical target volume (CTV), planning target volume (PTV) and OARs. All pixels in the extracted regions are assigned a unique teaching label to use as the training data for constructing the proposed system. Table 1 show the detailed information of all contours with its teaching label value and dose constraints. Here, there are five dose constraints for the IMRT: the maximum dose value (D_{max}), 1 cubic centimeter (D_{1cc}) of the dose, and 2%, 50% , 95% and 98% ($D_{2\%}$, D_{50}, $D_{95\%}$ and $D_{98\%}$) of the dose.

The IMRT for NPC treatment uses 7 dynamic beams whose orientations are 0, 51, 102, 153, 204, 255 and 306 [deg] around a patient. Each beam has 6 [MeV] energy. The target dose prescription was 70 Gy in 33 fractions (2.12 Gy per fraction and between 0.27 and 0.34 Gy for each beam). The 2D real dose image of each beam was constructed by using the parameters obtained from a radiotherapy treatment plan. Figure 1 shows an example of the real dose of each beam. The spatial resolution of the final dose distribution was 0.25×0.25 [cm].

2.2   System

Figure 2 shows the overview of the proposed system. The first phase of the proposed system is to predict the dose distribution delivered from each beam. The prediction system consists of seven modified U-net network, called

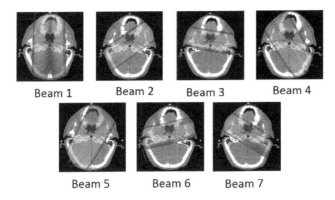

Fig. 1. An exemple of the dose of each beam.

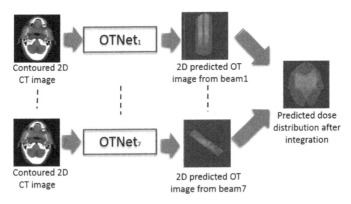

Fig. 2. The architecture of the proposed method.

"Optimal Treatment Networks (OTNets)" shown Fig. 3. Each OTNet is an encoder-decoder network. The encoder is composed of two networks which have the same architecture. The input of the first encoder network is the combination of the contours of tumors, that is, PTV, CTV and GTV while the second encoder is the contours of all OARs. The use of the two different networks aims to obtain more detailed features about tumor and OARs separately. Each network includes 42 convolutional layers for extracting the features of its target regions. The output of the encoder is the feature map of the input data. From the two feature maps of the tumors and OARs, the decoder network with deconvolutional layers generates the image of the 2D image of the optimal dose distribution delivered from the beam.

In the second phase, from multiple 2D dose images obtained from the seven OTNets, 2D dose distribution image for a patient is constructed by integrating all the dose images. Each pixel value of the predicted dose distribution image is the sum of all dose values obtained from multiple 2D dose images of the corresponding pixel. As a result, from all CT images of a patient, a 3D dose distribution image is created from all predicted 2D dose distribution images.

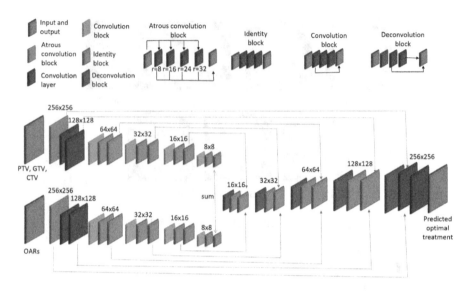

Fig. 3. The architecture of OTNet.

3   Experimental Results

To validate the applicability of the proposed method, we made experiments for predicting the dose distribution using our dataset composed of 80 patients. In the experiments, our dataset is divided into eight sub-datasets, each of which has 10 patient images. Using the sub-datasets, 8 fold cross validation is applied to evaluate the proposed system: 7 sub-datasets are used for training the proposed system while the rest sub-dataset is employed as a test data. Moreover, we use the manual dose distribution by radiation oncologists (MD) to compare it with the three methods.

3.1   Results

In the experiments, OTNet is compared with Mahmood et al. [8] (GAN) and Chen et al. [9] (ResNet101) methods. We downloaded and used directly the methods in [8,9] by using our database. The two networks predict the 2D optimal treatment images from contoured CT images.

When the contoured CT image in Fig. 4(a) is given as an input data, we obtain the dose distribution from the image predicted by OTNet (Fig. 4(c)), GAN (Fig. 4(d)) and ResNet101 (Fig. 4(e)), respectively. Figure 4(b) shows the manual dose distribution image obtained by radiation oncologists.

To compare with the three methods, a global 3D gamma analysis with 3%3mm and 4%4mm for $\gamma \leq 1$ was applied to evaluate the accuracy of OARs and tumor regions in the predicted dose distribution by the three methods. The calculated values of the mean pass rates of 3D gamma analysis are presented in Table 2.

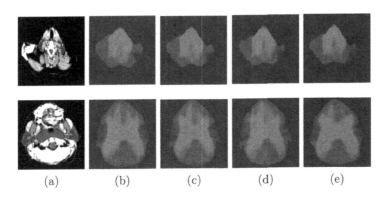

Fig. 4. Examples of (a) countoured CT image and its dose distribution obtained by (b) MD, (c) OTNet, (d) GAN and (e) ResNet101.

Table 2. Mean pass rates of 3D gamma analysis with 3%3mm and 4%4mm of OTNet, GAN and ResNet101.

	3%/3 mm (%)					4%/4 mm (%)				
	OTNet	GAN	p	ResNe101	p	OTNet	GAN	p	ResNe101	p
L/R TMJ	**90.2 ± 1.7**	88.5 ± 0.4	0.234	89.4 ± 1.1	0.147	**97.1 ± 0.6**	94.9 ± 0.3	0.193	95.2 ± 0.6	0.118
Optic chiasma	82.1 ± 0.9	86.4 ± 1.7	0.436	**88.0 ± 2.1**	0.247	93.6 ± 1.1	95.9 ± 2.3	0.294	**96.1 ± 0.7**	0.138
L/R Lens	**92.0 ± 4.8**	87.6 ± 1.7	0.449	89.1 ± 1.6	0.268	**98.1 ± 0.5**	94.1 ± 1.3	0.198	95.9 ± 2.9	0.165
Larynx	**79.1 ± 3.4**	76.1 ± 1.1	0.332	77.4 ± 2.1	0.141	**88.1 ± 1.7**	85.3 ± 1.2	0.302	86.9 ± 1.3	0.408
Temporal lobe	**85.5 ± 1.6**	82.7 ± 2.3	0.419	83.9 ± 0.3	0.231	**93.5 ± 0.6**	92.7 ± 1.6	0.118	93.1 ± 0.3	0.165
L/R Mandible	**80.1 ± 0.9**	77.3 ± 2.5	0.478	78.7 ± 1.2	0.114	**92.0 ± 0.4**	87.1 ± 2.0	0.271	86.2 ± 0.7	0.396
L/R optic nerve	**93.7 ± 4.6**	91.4 ± 5.1	0.314	91.8 ± 0.3	0.146	**97.8 ± 2.1**	93.9 ± 4.9	0.209	95.1 ± 1.0	0.343
L/R parotid gland	**88.4 ± 2.6**	86.7 ± 1.2	0.231	87.0 ± 0.5	0.117	**95.4 ± 2.8**	93.1 ± 0.6	0.191	93.8 ± 0.6	0.417
Brainstem	82.4 ± 2.1	**83.1 ± 0.7**	0.054	80.7 ± 0.8	0.124	89.9 ± 4.3	**91.2 ± 0.2**	0.115	88.9 ± 1.6	0.197
Spinal cord	**84.3 ± 5.2**	80.1 ± 2.3	0.429	80.9 ± 1.6	0.447	**94.2 ± 3.2**	91.2 ± 2.8	0.237	91.8 ± 0.9	0.232
PTV	**92.5 ± 7.3**	92.2 ± 4.1	0.105	92.2 ± 0.8	0.224	**99.7 ± 7.3**	98.1 ± 4.1	0.105	98.7 ± 0.8	0.093
GTV	**96.4 ± 3.5**	95.0 ± 1.4	0.290	95.5 ± 1.8	0.147	**97.8 ± 0.9**	95.0 ± 1.4	0.290	96.1 ± 2.8	0.143
CTV	**95.7 ± 3.9**	94.2 ± 2.1	0.184	94.5 ± 1.1	0.228	**99.0 ± 1.6**	98.7 ± 1.4	0.184	98.9 ± 4.1	0.367

Table 3. MAE_{DVH} of each region by OTNet, GAN and ResNet101.

Contours	OTNet	GAN	ResNet101	Contours	OTNet	GAN	ResNet101
L/R TMJ	**1.2 ± 0.5**	1.4 ± 0.6	1.4 ± 0.2	L/R parotid gland	**1.4 ± 1.5**	1.8 ± 0.3	1.7 ± 0.8
Optic chiasma	1.7 ± 0.3	1.9 ± 0.6	**1.3 ± 1.1**	Brainstem	1.5 ± 1.1	**1.2 ± 0.9**	1.6 ± 0.2
L/R Lens	**1.4 ± 0.8**	1.9 ± 0.4	1.6 ± 0.7	Spinal cord	**1.3 ± 0.6**	1.4 ± 1.2	1.4 ± 0.7
Larynx	**1.9 ± 0.7**	2.6 ± 0.8	2.2 ± 1.3	PTV	**0.9 ± 0.5**	1.2 ± 1.0	1.1 ± 1.3
Temporal lobe	**0.9 ± 0.4**	1.7 ± 0.1	1.2 ± 0.6	GTV	**0.8 ± 0.7**	1.0 ± 0.7	1.0 ± 0.8
L/R Mandible	**1.2 ± 0.9**	1.3 ± 0.8	1.3 ± 0.9	CTV	**0.7 ± 0.9**	1.2 ± 0.8	0.9 ± 1.4
L/R optic nerve	**1.0 ± 0.6**	1.5 ± 0.2	1.4 ± 0.5				

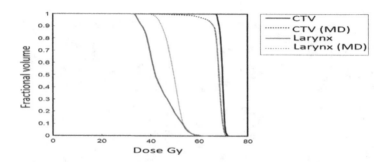

Fig. 5. DVH of OTNet vs MD

In addition, we calculated the difference between the predicted cumulative dose volume histograms (DVHs) of each method and MD. Here, DVH indicates the dose value per fractional volume of the target region. Moreover, the difference between two DVHs is formulated by mean absolute error of DVH:

$$MAE_{DVH} = \frac{1}{m} \sum_{k=1}^{m} \frac{1}{n} \sum_{j=1}^{n} |D_p(j)_{k\%} - D_g(j)_{k\%}|, \qquad (1)$$

where m is the number of DVH bins separated by 0.01 Gy, k is the dose volume index of DVH, j is the 2D dose distribution image of the target region, n is the total number of images. $D_p(j)_{k\%}$ and $D_g(j)_{k\%}$ are the predicted and MD doses value at $k\%$ volume of the pixel of the jth image, respectively.

Figure 5 shows the examples of the predicted DVHs for CTV and Larynx of OTNet and MD to which the differences to MD are the minimum and maximum among other contours.

3.2   Discussion

As shown in Table 2, except the brainstem and optic chiasma, the mean pass rates of 3D gamma of OTNet is higher than those of GAN and ResNet101 for most of OARs. Similarly, from Table 3, MAE of OTNet is the smallest among the three methods except brainstem and optic chiasma. In addition, in the both cases of the global 3D gamma analysis with 3%/3mm and 4%/4mm, the mean pass rates of all regions with OTNet is the highest among three methods. To compare OTNet with the other two methods, the statistical analysis is performed with paired t-tests (p-value(P) < 0.05). However, the t-test indicates that OTNet is not significantly different from the two comparison methods for all OARs. From the 3D gamma analysis, OTNet predicts almost the same dose distribution as MD compared with the two comparison methods.

From these results, we conclude that our proposed method, especially OTNet, can predict the dose distribution with a good performance. In addition, we find that OTNet results a high accuracy for small volume of OARs, such as left and right Lens, except the brainstem and optic chiasma. This may due to the strategy that we used in our network OTNet. By training Tumors and OARs regions separately, the network train the dataset with more detailed information. However, due to the shape of optic chiasma and brainstem, its proximity to the tumor regions and high dose value, OTNet predict these regions with low performance compared to the other methods. Since our network is a simple network, a deeper and complex architecture, like ResNet101 and GAN, is needed to improve the results of complex volume regions.

4   Conclusion

In this paper, we proposed a new CNN, OTNet, which predicts the dose distribution for a patient from contoured CT images. In the proposed method, the optimal dose distribution of each beam is estimated from contoured CT images. The dose distribution for a patient is obtained by integrating the dose images of all the beams. From the experimental results, our proposed network, OTNet, can predict the dose distribution reliably and accurately compared with the conventional methods.

In this work, we focused on the prediction of dose prediction without considering dose constraints of OARs and tumor regions. One of our future works is to train OTNet with an optimization function of dose to improve the prediction accuracy of dose constrain of predicted dose distribution.

Acknowledgement. This work was supported by JST CREST Grant Number JPMJCR1786, JSPS KAKENHI Grant Number 19H04139, and JIUN Corporation.

References

1. Mendenhall, W.M., Amdur, R.J., Palta, J.R.: Intensity-modulated radiotherapy in the standard management of head and neck cancer: promises and pitfalls. J. Clin. Oncol. **24**(17), 2618–2623 (2006)
2. Oelfke, U., Bortfeld, T.: Inverse planning for photon and proton beams. Med. Dosim. **26**(2), 113–124 (2001)
3. Nelms, B.E., Robinson, G., Markham, J., et al.: Variation in external beam treatment plan quality: an inter-institutional study of planners and planning systems. Pract. Radiat. Oncol. **2**(4), 296–305 (2012)
4. Xhaferllari, I., Wong, E., Karl, B., Michael, L., Jeff, Z.C.: Automated IMRT planning with regional optimization using planning scripts. J. Appl. Clin. Med. Phys. **14**(1), 176–191 (2013)
5. Folkerts, M., et al.: Knowledge-based automatic treatment planning for prostate IMRT using 3-dimensional dose prediction and threshold-based optimization: SU-E-FS2-06. Med. Phys. **44**(6), 2728 (2017)
6. Long, J., Shelhamer, E., Darrell, T.: Fully convolutional networks for semantic segmentation. In: Proceedings of the IEEE Conference on Computer Vision and Pattern Recognition, pp. 3431–3440 (2015)

7. Zhen, X., et al.: Deep convolutional neural network with transfer learning for rectum toxicity prediction in cervical cancer radiotherapy: a feasibility study. Phys. Med. Biol. **62**(21), 8246 (2017)

8. Mahmood, R., Babier, A., McNiven, A., Diamant, A., Chan, T.C.: Automated treatment planning in radiation therapy using generative adversarial networks. arXiv preprint arXiv:1807.06489 (2018)

9. Chen, X., Men, K., Li, Y., Yi, J., Dai, J.: A feasibility study on an automated method to generate patient-specific dose distributions for radiotherapy using deep learning. Med. phys. **46**(1), 56–64 (2019)

DeepMCDose: A Deep Learning Method for Efficient Monte Carlo Beamlet Dose Calculation by Predictive Denoising in MR-Guided Radiotherapy

Ryan Neph$^{(\boxtimes)}$ ⓘ, Yangsibo Huang, Youming Yang, and Ke Sheng

University of California – Los Angeles, Los Angeles, CA 90095, USA
ryanneph@ucla.edu

Abstract. The next great leap toward improving treatment of cancer with radiation will require the combined use of online adaptive and magnetic resonance guided radiation therapy techniques with automatic X-ray beam orientation selection. Unfortunately, by uniting these advancements, we are met with a substantial expansion in the required dose information and consequential increase to the overall computational time imposed during radiation treatment planning, which cannot be handled by existing techniques for accelerating Monte Carlo dose calculation. We propose a deep convolutional neural network approach that unlocks new levels of acceleration and accuracy with regards to post-processed Monte Carlo dose results by relying on data-driven learned representations of low-level beamlet dose distributions instead of more limited filter-based denoising techniques that only utilize the information in a single dose input. Our method uses parallel U-Net branches acting on three input channels before mixing latent understanding to produce noise-free dose predictions. Our model achieves a normalized mean absolute error of only 0.106% compared with the ground truth dose contrasting the 25.7% error of the under sampled MC dose fed into the network at prediction time. Our model's per-beamlet prediction time is ~220 ms, including Monte Carlo simulation and network prediction, with substantial additional acceleration expected from batched processing and combination with existing Monte Carlo acceleration techniques. Our method shows promise toward enabling clinical practice of advanced treatment technologies.

Keywords: Radiation dose prediction · Deep learning · CNN · Monte Carlo

1 Introduction

Magnetic resonance guided radiotherapy (MRgRT) is an innovation that asserts dominance over traditional CT-guided radiotherapy with respect to the offered soft tissue contrast and imaging flexibility. Such innovations in the pre-treatment imaging and the online image-guided contexts have enabled enhanced precision in the treatment of inconspicuous and moving lesions. The difficulty of widespread adoption of MRgRT is in part due to the complicating behavior of charged particles (electrons) in the

© Springer Nature Switzerland AG 2019
D. Nguyen et al. (Eds.): AIRT 2019, LNCS 11850, pp. 137–145, 2019.
https://doi.org/10.1007/978-3-030-32486-5_17

presence of a moderate to strong magnetic field. The result is a non-negligible perturbation to the more typical dose distributions observed without a strong magnetic field. Great effort has been invested in acceleration of deterministic dose calculation, including the works of Chen [1], Neylon [2] and most recently Neph [3] which emphasize efficient GPU implementation. However, the effects of a strong magnetic field fundamentally invalidate the assumptions made by these heavily relied upon deterministic dose calculation algorithms, leaving us instead with highly the accurate and flexible, but comparably less efficient Monte Carlo (MC) dose simulation technique.

The intersection of MRgRT with other advanced clinical techniques presents a serious challenge with respect to the capabilities of existing MC dose calculation tools. Online adaptive radiotherapy (OART) deviates from the clinical standard by both re-imaging and re-optimizing RT treatment plans prior to each daily radiation delivery. The outcome of OART is increased delivery precision and improved patient outcome but is commonly rendered computationally intractable given the insufficient speed of both the dose calculation and plan optimization stages. Additionally, the innovation of beam orientation optimization (BOO) increases plan quality while simplifying the planning effort. However, BOO imparts a substantial requirement on the compulsory dose data that is calculated prior to the start of planning. Current clinical practice with human pre-selection of around 10 static beams necessitates calculation of *planning* dose distributions for a few thousand individual beamlets. By comparison, joint optimization of beam orientations and their fluence maps performed by 4pi treatment planning, considers 1162 candidate beam orientations and requires calculation of dose for hundreds of thousands of beamlets consequently.

It is well understood that each of these techniques offer significant and complementary improvements to the treatment planning process and quality of patient care. However, the convergence of their practice imposes formidable challenges on the dose calculation component of the planning process; namely that we must simultaneously pivot to using more accurate methods, which can handle EREs, while greatly increasing the efficiency to handle significant increases to the amount of prerequisite data. In summary, we must find a way to get the accuracy benefits of MC dose simulation while accelerating its computation time beyond that which is possible using any existing MC acceleration techniques.

Previous work on accelerating MC simulation has investigated the use of denoising algorithms applied to under sampled (noisy) MC dose. Deasy [4] used a wavelet coefficient thresholding approach to denoising on a slice-by-slice basis. Kawrakow [5] presents a 3D implementation of locally adaptive Savitzky-Golay filtering that selects the anisotropic filter window size by means of a locally supported chi-square test, limiting the effect of systematic bias. Fippel [6] proposed an optimization approach including both dose fidelity and smoothness regularization terms. Miao [7] investigated the use of an adaptive denoising approach modeling the dose in terms of heat transport and used anisotropic diffusion to achieve smoothed distributions. El Naqa [8] used a hybrid median filtering approach which adapts the filter to the local content of the dose distribution to more effectively tradeoff the benefits of mean- and median-based denoising.

This existing work places an emphasis on only moderately under sampled dose suggesting their incapacity to robustly and accurately denoise dose with anything beyond this modest level of noise or in heterogeneous geometries. El Naqa [9] judges that "uncertainties of greater than 5% are probably too large" for producing clinically usable treatment plans, and that "maximum error of denoised distributions can still be large for raw MC uncertainties of 3%", indicating observed errors up to 15% in these cases.

Our contributions focus on meeting this need. We harness a successful Deep Learning model architecture, U-Net [10], to perform concurrent denoising and prediction of *noise-free* MR-guided beamlet dose from an extremely noisy (and cheap to simulate) version of the MC beamlet dose for the given geometry. Additionally, we show that our model performs well in previously unseen patient geometries for a given anatomical region such as the head and neck, supporting our expectation of its generalizability for clinical use. We further note that while our model contributes a significant level of acceleration to the task of very-large-scale (VLS) dose calculation, it remains fully compatible with existing MC acceleration techniques such as GPU-based simulation and variance reduction, reinforcing its promise for clinical application.

2 Methods

We present a novel technique for accelerated calculation of X-ray beamlet dose from highly under sampled (noisy) Monte Carlo simulation. Our model incorporates the widely successful U-NET CNN architecture to learn the actual dose distribution of an X-ray beamlet, including perturbations resulting from EREs in the presence of an MR-induced magnetic field.

Our model is composed of three independent U-Net branches, each with 4 hierarchical levels, that learn a latent representation of each of 3 input channels: under sampled dose, MC X-ray fluence, and CT geometry. Channel-specific latent

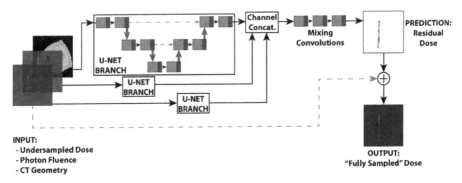

Fig. 1. Monte Carlo dose prediction network architecture. Parallel U-Net branches process each input channel independently. Concatenation and mixing of latent representations produces predicted residual dose. Residual and under sampled doses are summed, giving prediction of fully sampled dose.

representations are mixed in a series of fully convolutional layers which preserve the original data dimensionality and produce a prediction of the residual between the input (noisy) and ground-truth dose. Adding the residual and input dose gives the predicted noise-free dose. A summary of the network architecture is shown in Fig. 1.

2.1   Monte Carlo Dose Simulation

A general purpose, CPU-based Monte Carlo particle simulation toolkit, Geant4 v10.4 [11, 12], was used obtain the under sampled and fully sampled beamlet dose distributions as well as the X-ray fluence for each beamlet configuration. A single instance of the fully sampled dose was simulated by tracking 18 million X-rays from a point source 100 cm away from the beamlet's isocenter in a uniformly diverging square field. Ten under sampled doses were additionally simulated by instead tracking 500 X-rays each in the same manner. Each beamlet was modeled with an identical histogram-based energy distribution matching that of a clinical 6MV Bremsstrahlung spectrum. To understand the applicability of our approach to MRgRT, we configured a static 1.5T magnetic field, oriented in parallel to the rotation axis of the X-ray source around the treatment isocenter; this geometry matches that of existing MRgRT treatment devices such as the Elekta Unity©.

To standardize the amount of noise present in the under sampled MC dose distributions, we incrementally simulated beamlet dose for 50 randomly selected beamlets in the testing dataset, monitoring the normalized mean absolute error (NMAE) compared with the fully sampled dose until it reached a threshold of 25%. For the fully sampled dose, we selected an average statistical uncertainty during MC simulation of less than 0.1% as the threshold. To maintain these average qualities of dose, the under sampled inputs and fully sampled ground truths were simulated using 500 and 18 million X-rays as described earlier in this section.

2.2   Dataset Construction

Beamlets configurations consisted of beam azimuth (gantry angle), isocenter coordinates, and beamlet position within the beam. The parameters of the beamlet configuration were selected randomly to ensure diversity in both the training and testing datasets. Ten head and neck (H&N) CT volumes were retrospectively collected from UCLA's database of radiation treatments and resampled to have an isotropic voxel size of 2.5 mm^3. Six of the patients were reserved for training and the remaining four for unbiased testing of the trained model. We are careful to test on patients that are previously unseen during the training process so an unbiased evaluation of the model generalizability to new patients can be reported. For each *training* and *testing* patient, an average of 865 and 415 beamlet configurations were randomly sampled, respectively.

A single data example was created by pairing each three-channel input with the fully sampled dose for a specific beamlet configuration. To augment the dataset with extra data examples, rather than randomly generate additional beamlet configurations and perform additional, and expensive, MC simulation of the fully sampled (ground-truth) dose, we recognized that each under sampled simulation of dose is an independent and identically distributed (IID) stochastic observation of the fully sampled dose. This allowed us to pair a single fully sampled dose with multiple (currently 10) independent under sampled inputs. This augmentation technique is like the addition of zero-mean gaussian noise used more commonly in natural image domains, except that we can sample directly from the true noise model by use of MC simulation. After augmentation, our training and testing datasets contained 155,940 and 49,770 examples, respectively.

Our model was trained for 150 epochs ($\sim$ 183,000 iterations) in a data-parallel manner across four NVIDIA GTX Titan X graphics processing units (GPUs). Training time was approximately 18 h, though the greatest reduction to the loss function was seen after just a few hours. Batch normalization and ReLU operations were used between each convolutional layer.

2.3   Experiment Design

To assess the accuracy of the predicted beamlet dose results, we computed the NMAE across every voxel of every beamlet in the testing dataset. To provide physical meaning to this metric, each voxel of the predicted beamlet dose was normalized to the corresponding beamlet-maximum dose, obtained from the fully sampled MC dose volume. We also computed spatial gamma index maps, which indicate the dosimetric accuracy of voxels by combining the dose difference and distance-to-agreement metrics, for each of a pre-determined set of gamma criteria. Readers are referred to [13] for a complete description of the gamma index. Voxels with a gamma index of less than or equal to 1.0, are regarded as *passing* the gamma test, while those with indices in excess of 1.0 are failing, which generally indicate regions of degraded dosimetric accuracy. Our results show *passing* voxels in blue and failing voxels in red, with white indicating the division between the two classifications. Gamma maps are provided for the 0.2%/ 0.2 mm, 0.5%/0.5 mm, and 1%/1 mm gamma criteria. In our reporting of the results, the NMAE was masked to reduce the bias of less-important voxels with very-low dose. Our masking operation excludes those voxels having both ground truth and predicted normalized dose under 10%, which ensures that both the actual dose and any possible false predictions of dose are low enough to be ignored in most cases.

3   Results

In our experiment, where the accuracy of the under sampled MC dose and the deep model predicted dose were compared with respect to the ground truth, a NMAE of 25.7% before prediction and 0.106% after were observed. Prediction time for a single beamlet was approximately 220 ms, including both the MC simulation and network prediction steps, while the time to produce a single fully sampled beamlet dose was approximately 380 s on average. Figure 2 shows the under sampled (input), network predicted, and fully sampled (ground truth) dose for a single beamlet passing through a large air cavity within the patient's mouth, where EREs are expected and observed. Figure 3 additionally shows the gamma index maps for the beamlet shown in Fig. 2. Darks blue voxels indicate those that easily pass the gamma test for the imposed criteria (index much less than 1.0). Dark red voxels conversely indicate dramatic failure by the gamma criteria (index much greater than 1.0. Lighter shades of each color, and white indicate voxels that lie near the threshold with index value equal to 1.0.

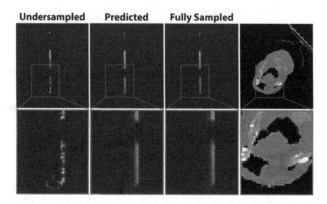

Fig. 2. Comparison of under sampled, predicted, and fully sampled (ground truth) dose for one beamlet. Bottom row shows close-up of soft tissue-air interfaces where EREs are visible. (Color figure online)

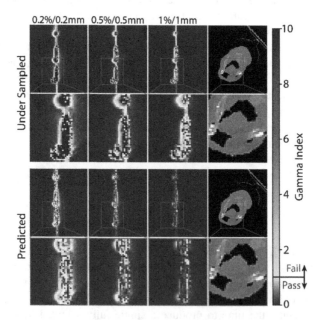

Fig. 3. Gamma maps for one under sampled and predicted beamlet dose distribution compared to the ground truth (fully sampled dose). Red voxels indicate large disagreement while white and blue indicate passing for the referenced gamma criterion. Close-up views given under each. (Color figure online)

4 Discussion

We observe from the analysis of dosimetric accuracy between the under sampled dose and the deep network prediction that a substantial improvement in the beamlet dose accuracy is achieved despite imparting less than 200 ms for the additional prediction step. Indicated by the reduction of NMAE for the testing dataset, the accuracy improvement between the under sampled dose and the predicted dose is greater than two orders of magnitude. Without a dedicated analysis of the resulting effects on the treatment planning process, it is difficult to conclude from this study whether the observed accuracy is sufficient for clinical use. However, from the conclusions drawn in [9] we show that our dose prediction model outperforms existing denoising methods with NMAE below 0.2% (improvement ratio of 242) compared to the best performing method of [4] achieving an improvement ratio of only 4.5, corresponding to a NMAE of approximately 1.21% (MSE improvement ratio of 4.5 for the 6.6% uncertainty input) for the H&N evaluation. This improvement is evident despite starting with much noisier dose inputs (input NMAE of more than 25% in our case, compared with up to 6.6% MC uncertainty selected to evaluate the methods of [4] in [9]).

Furthermore, investigating the predicted dose distribution in Fig. 2 and the corresponding gamma index maps in Fig. 3 clearly show the advantage of our deep learning-based approach in both the global denoising and the local ERE prediction tasks. For example, the under sampled dose in Fig. 2 displays a *dose loop* which is commonly observed in noisy MR-guide MC results but is not representative of the expectation obtained by full sampling to a low uncertainty. For these situations, where local filtering approaches tend to fail to distinguish this low probability stochastic event from the true beamlet structure, our model can disambiguate the two and harness the information to produce a more realistic prediction. Moreover, the qualitative differences in the gamma maps of Fig. 3 clearly demonstrate the global predictive performance of our model, where the fraction of red voxels is substantially reduced between the under sampled and predicted dose distributions.

Like the denoising methods presented in [4–8], our model also benefits from batched evaluation for both the MC simulation and especially the GPU-based model prediction steps. The runtimes reported in Sect. 3 were limited to computation of a single beamlet dose distribution without including the benefits of batched processing. With even a modest availability of GPU hardware and GPU-enabled MC simulation tools, we expect that parallel processing will greatly improve the average per-beamlet processing time well beyond that which is required of online adaptive MRgRT. Further investigation of the limits of acceleration that can be achieved and the benefits to the actual process of treatment plan optimization using predicted beamlet dose distributions are planned for future work.

5 Conclusions

We have demonstrated the success of our novel deep learning-based approach to beamlet-scale Monte Carlo dose denoising in terms of the computational time and accuracy improvements. Our technique differs from existing attempts at MC dose denoising in that it: has been evaluated for use in MRgRT where EREs induce local perturbations to the simpler no-magnetic-field X-ray dose distribution, is applicable to substantially noisier dose input resulting from fewer MC-simulated particles, and benefits from efficient deep CNN prediction while maintaining compatibility with existing MC acceleration techniques. By testing our model performance with patient geometries that were not used during model training, our method shows generalizability to new patients, and normalized mean absolute beamlet dose errors of 0.106% on average, compared with the 25.7% error observed by directly using the under sampled dose. This performance is demonstrated while reducing the dose calculation time by over two orders of magnitude compared with fully sampled MC beamlet dose. Our method shows promise in enabling clinical use of adaptive online MRgRT for automatically planned treatments.

References

1. Chen, Q., Chen, M., Lu, W.: Ultrafast convolution/superposition using tabulated and exponential kernels on GPU. Med. Phys. **38**(3), 1150–1161 (2011). https://doi.org/10.1118/1.3551996
2. Neylon, J., et al.: A nonvoxel-based dose convolution/superposition algorithm optimized for scalable GPU architectures. Med. Phys. **41**(10), 101711 (2014). https://doi.org/10.1118/1.4895822
3. Neph, R., Ouyang, C., Neylon, J., Yang, Y.M., Sheng, K.: Parallel beamlet dose calculation via beamlet contexts in a distributed Multi-GPU Framework. Med. Phys. (2019). https://doi.org/10.1002/mp.13651
4. Deasy, J.O., Wickerhauser, M.V., Picard, M.: Accelerating Monte Carlo simulations of radiation therapy dose distributions using wavelet threshold de-noising. Med. Phys. **29**(10), 2366–2373 (2002). https://doi.org/10.1118/1.1508112
5. Kawrakow, I.: On the de-noising of Monte Carlo calculated dose distributions. Phys. Med. Biol. **47**(17), 304 (2002). https://doi.org/10.1088/0031-9155/47/17/304
6. Fippel, M., Nüsslin, F.: Smoothing Monte Carlo calculated dose distributions by iterative reduction of noise. Phys. Med. Biol. **48**(10), 1289–1304 (2003). https://doi.org/10.1088/0031-9155/48/10/304
7. Miao, B., Jeraj, R., Bao, S., Mackie, T.R.: Adaptive anisotropic diffusion filtering of Monte Carlo dose distributions. Phys. Med. Biol. **48**(17), 2767–2781 (2003). https://doi.org/10.1088/0031-9155/48/17/303
8. El Naqa, I., Deasy, J.O., Vicic, M.: Locally adaptive denoising of Monte Carlo dose distributions via hybrid median filtering. In: IEEE Nuclear Science Symposium, pp. 2703–2706 (2003). ISBN 0-7803-8257-9
9. El Naqa, I., et al.: A comparison of Monte Carlo dose calculation denoising techniques. Phys. Med. Biol. **50**(5), 909–922 (2005). https://doi.org/10.1088/0031-9155/50/5/014
10. Ronneberger, O., Fischer, P., Brox, T.: U-Net: convolutional networks for biomedical image segmentation. In: Navab, N., Hornegger, J., Wells, W.M., Frangi, A.F. (eds.) MICCAI 2015. LNCS, vol. 9351, pp. 234–241. Springer, Cham (2015). https://doi.org/10.1007/978-3-319-24574-4_28
11. Agostinelli, S., et al.: GEANT4—a simulation toolkit. Nuclear Instrum. Methods Phys. Res. Sect. A Accel. Spectrom. Detect. Assoc. Equip. **506**(3), 250–303 (2003). https://doi.org/10.1016/S0168-9002(03)01368-8

12. Allison, J., et al.: Recent developments in GEANT4. Nuclear Instrum. Methods Phys. Res. Sect. A Accel. Spectrom. Detect. Assoc. Equip. **835**, 186–225 (2016). https://doi.org/10.1016/j.nima.2016.06.125
13. Low, D.A., Harms, W.B., Mutic, S., Purdy, J.A.: A technique for the quantitative evaluation of dose distributions. Med. Phys. **25**(5), 656–661 (1998). https://doi.org/10.1118/1.598248

UC-GAN for MR to CT Image Synthesis

Haitao Wu[1,2], Xiling Jiang[3], and Fucang Jia[1,2(✉)]

[1] Shenzhen Institutes of Advanced Technology,
Chinese Academy of Sciences, Shenzhen, China
fc.jia@siat.ac.cn
[2] Shenzhen College of Advanced Technology,
University of Chinese Academy of Sciences, Shenzhen, China
[3] College of Oral Medicine, Chifeng University, Chifeng, China

Abstract. Accurate MR-to-CT synthesis plays an important role in MRI-only radiotherapy treatment planning. In medical image synthesis, the cycle-generative adversarial network (CycleGAN) is becoming an influential method, however, its image quality of synthesis is not optimal yet. In this study, we proposed a new learning method named U-Net-CycleGAN (UC-GAN) to generate synthetic CT (sCT) image for MRI-only radiation treatment planning, which integrated an improved U-Net concept into the original CycleGAN framework. After experimental comparison, The MAE value and PSNR of our UC-GAN model are 76.7 ± 4.5 and 46.1 ± 1.5, respectively, which are statistics significantly better than the 94.0 ± 4.3 (MAE) and 45.1 ± 1.5 (PSNR) of the original CycleGAN model. The results of our quantitative evaluation show that the UC-GAN model can synthesize a CT image closer to the reference real CT image with better performance.

Keywords: U-Net · CycleGAN · Image synthesis · MR-to-CT

1 Introduction

Radiotherapy treatment planning requires a magnetic resonance (MR) volume for segmentation of tumor volume and organs at risk (OAR), as well as a spatially corresponding computed tomography (CT) volume for dose planning. Separate acquisition of these volumes is time-consuming, costly, and a burden to the patient. Furthermore, voxel-wise spatial alignment between MR and CT images may be compromised, requiring accurate registration of MR and CT volumes. Hence, to circumvent separate CT acquisition, a range of methods have been proposed for MR-only radiotherapy treatment planning in which a substitute or synthetic CT image is derived from the available MR image [1].

Medical image synthesis is defined as the generation of realistic images through learning models. From a technical perspective, image synthesis can be achieved from a generative model (e.g., from noise) or a cross-modality adaptation model (e.g., from MRI to CT) [2]. Our work is mostly related to the cross-modality image synthesis approaches, in which a synthetic image in target imaging modality is synthesized from a real image in source imaging modality. Historically, cross-modality image synthesis methods can be ascribed to three categories (1) atlas-based methods, (2) voxel-based

© Springer Nature Switzerland AG 2019
D. Nguyen et al. (Eds.): AIRT 2019, LNCS 11850, pp. 146–153, 2019.
https://doi.org/10.1007/978-3-030-32486-5_18

methods, and (3) deep learning based methods. In atlas-based methods, a set of one or multiple co-registered MR-CT images are deformably registered to a patient's MR image [3]. The resulting transformation can then be applied on the CT-atlas to generate the sCT image. Atlas-based approaches can be time-consuming, particularly when the atlases are large, and often fail if the patient has very different anatomy from what is represented by the atlas [2].

Voxel-based methods convert individual MR voxel intensities to HU values using bulk density assignments or machine learning models. Bulk density techniques assign the patient's electron density either to water or to pre-defined electron densities within selected MR-segmented tissue types [4]. These methods may lead to dose discrepancies and often have limited value in generating positioning reference images. Machine learning methods use paired MR-CT images to train models that associate MR intensities with HU values. It is challenging for models to distinguish air from bone in conventional MR images as both tissues exhibit weak signals due to their small T2 values. Some learning methods required manual bone segmentation [6] in conventional MR images or require acquisition of specialized MR sequences like ultrashort echo time sequences [7] for separating bone and air. Some methods used multiple MR images acquired with additional sequences designed to distinguish different tissue types [8]. Adding sequences can increase workload and extend scan time [2].

Herein, we focus on the third family - deep learning based image synthesis methods. Van Nguyen et al. proposed a location-sensitive deep synthesis method to utilize the both intensity and spatial information between modalities during training stage [5]. Sevetlidis et al. proposed a deep encoder-decoder network using a patch-based learning fashion [9]. Xiang et al. proposed a deep embedding convolutional neural network (CNN), which utilize the intermediate feature maps between MR and CT scans [10]. The generative adversarial network (GAN) [11] was improved by Nie et al. to deal with context-aware information in generating CT images from MR images [12].

Recently, many methods have been proposed to train image-to-image translation CNNs with unpaired natural images, namely DualGAN [13] and CycleGAN [14]. Like the methods proposed in [12, 15, 16], these CNNs translate an image from one domain to another domain. Different from these methods, the loss function in the training process is completely dependent on the overall quality of the integrated image, and the quality of the integrated image is determined by a network of confrontation discriminators. In order to prevent synthetic CNN from generating images that look real but are almost indistinguishable from the input image, it is necessary to enhance the loop consistency. That is, an additional CNN is trained to convert the synthesized image back to the original domain, and the difference between the reconstructed image and the original image is added as a regular term during training.

In this paper, we propose a new approach that combines an improved U-Net network [15] with a conventional CycleGAN model [14], and experiments have shown that our method got better synthesis performance. We have proved that the current deep learning model can continue to improve in the field of image synthesis.

2   Method

The proposed UC-GAN model consists of a generation phase and a discriminating phase (as shown in Fig. 1). For a given pair of MRI images and their corresponding CT images, CT images are used as deep learning targets for MRI images. Intra-subject registration was performed for each pair of CT and MRI images. Due to the small mismatch between the rigidly registered MRI and CT, and the difference in image properties between the two modalities, the constraints imposed on the MRI-to-CT conversion model are very low. In order to solve this problem, a CycleGAN containing inverse transform is introduced to capture the relationship between CT and MRI images, and the MRI-CT conversion model is inversely supervised. Due to the contrast between MRI and CT, high frequency features can be easily extracted from previous hidden layers. At the same time, the structural information of the MRI does not necessarily correspond to the structural information of the CT. Therefore, the MR-to-CT conversion is full shot. To further modify this to a bijective mapping, we introduced a U-Net architecture to combine and refine the high frequency features of the previous hidden layer and the anatomical (low frequency) features of the deep hidden layer. In the generation phase, the extracted training MRI patch slice is input into the generator (MRI-to-CT) to obtain a prediction CT of the same size, called sCT (fake CT).

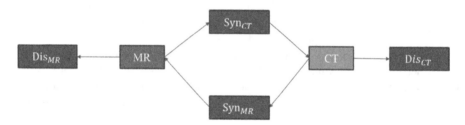

Fig. 1. The CycleGAN model consists of a forward loop and a backward loop. In the forward loop, Syn_{CT} synthesizes the CT image from the input MR image, Syn_{MR} reconstructs the input MR image from the synthesized image, and Dis_{CT} discriminates the real and synthesized CT images. In the reverse loop, Syn_{MR} synthesizes the MR image from the input CT image, Syn_{CT} reconstructs the input CT image from the synthesized image, and Dis_{MR} discriminates the real and synthesized MR images.

The adversarial goals of the synthesis and discriminator networks are reflected in their loss functions. The discriminator Dis_{CT} aims to predict the label 1 for real CT images and the label 0 for synthesized CT images. Hence, the discriminator Dis_{CT} tries to minimize

$$\mathcal{L}_{CT} = (1 - Dis_{CT}(I_{CT}))^2 + Dis_{CT}(Syn_{CT}(I_{MR}))^2 \tag{1}$$

for MR images I_{MR} and CT images I_{CT}. At the same time, synthesis network Syn_{CT} tries to maximize this loss by synthesizing images that cannot be distinguished from real CT images [17].

Similarly, the discriminator Dis_{MR} aims to predict the label 1 for real MR images and the label 0 for synthesized MR images. Hence, the loss function for MR synthesis that Dis_{MR} aims to minimize and Syn_{MR} aims to maximize is defined as

$$\mathcal{L}_{MR} = (1 - Dis_{MR}(I_{MR}))^2 + Dis_{MR}(Syn_{MR}(I_{CT}))^2 \tag{2}$$

To enforce bidirectional cycle consistency during training, additional loss terms are defined as the difference between original and reconstructed images,

$$\mathcal{L}_{Cycle} = \|Syn_{MR}(Syn_{CT}(I_{MR})) - I_{MR}\|_1 + \|Syn_{CT}(Syn_{MR}(I_{CT})) - I_{CT}\|_1 \tag{3}$$

During training, this term is weighted by a parameter λ and added to the loss functions for Syn_{CT} and Syn_{MR} [17].

2.1 Generator

The whole structure of the generator is based on the 2D DCNN model proposed by Han et al. [15]. The model can be seen as consisting of two main parts: an encoding part (left half) and a decoding part (right half). The encoding part behaves as traditional

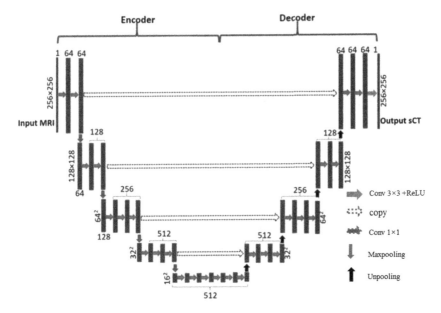

Fig. 2. The overall structure of the generator network. Each yellow arrow represents a (3×3) convolutional operation (with a rectified linear unit as the activation function). Each green arrow represents a Maxpooling operation, and each black arrow represents a unpooling operation. Each white arrow represents a duplicate operation. The top of each blue box provides the 2D image size and depth (number of channels) from the feature map for each convolutional operation. The red arrow indicates the last 1×1 convolution operation that generated the output sCT prediction. (Color figure online)

CNNs that learn to extract a hierarchy of increasingly complex features from an input MR image [15]. The decoding part transforms the features and gradually reconstructs the sCT prediction from low to high resolution. The final output of the network is a 2D image with the same size as the input image. A key innovation from Ronneberger et al. [18] that we borrow here is to introduce direct connections (shown as white arrows in Fig. 2) across the encoding part and the decoding part so that high resolution features from the first part can be used as extra inputs for the convolutional layers in the second part [15].

2.2   Evaluation

Real and synthesized CT images were compared using the mean absolute error (MAE)

$$MAE = \frac{1}{N}\sum_{i=1}^{N} |I_{CT}(i) - Syn_{CT}(I_{MR}(i))|, \tag{4}$$

where i iterates over aligned voxels in the real and synthesized CT images. Note that this was based on the prior alignment of I_{MR} and I_{CT}. In addition, agreement was evaluated using the peak-signal-to-noise-ratio (PSNR) as proposed in [12, 15] as

$$PSNR = 20\log_{10}\frac{4095}{MSE}, \tag{5}$$

Where MSE is the mean-squared error, i.e. $\frac{1}{N}\sum_{i=1}^{N} (I_{CT}(i) - Syn_{CT}(I_{MR}(i)))^2$. The MAE and PSNR were computed within a head region mask determined in both the CT and MR that excludes any surrounding air [17].

3   Experiments and Results

In order to test our synthesis method, we applied the proposed method to brain MR and CT images. We collected the paired brain MR and CT data from 6 patients. Each CT or MR volume involved more than 222 2D axial image slices. These were resampled to 256×256 in 256-grayscale and uniformly distributed by $[-1000, 1000]$ HU for CT data and whole HU for MR data. For each patient we obtained 222 2D slices of MR and CT.

For training, we augmented each patient's slices data with random transforms [19]:

- *Flip:* Batch data were horizontally flipped with 0.5 probability.
- *Translation:* Batch data were randomly cropped to size 256×256 from padded 286×286.
- *Rotation:* Batch data were rotated by $r \in [-5, 5]$ degrees.

We choose the leave-one-out method for experiments. Each experiment five patient's data-augmentation dataset were selected to be the training set, and the remaining patient's original dataset was used as the test set, and the experiment was performed using the conventional CycleGAN and our proposed method separately. We use the default value of $\lambda = 10$ to weigh cycle consistency loss. The model was trained using Adam [20] for 100 epochs with a fixed learning rate of 0.0002, and 100 epochs in which the learning rate was linearly reduced to zero. Model training took 120 h on a single NVIDIA Tesla V100 GPU. MR to CT synthesis with a trained model took around 10 s.

We compared the proposed method to the conventional CycleGAN. The results are shown in Table 1.

Table 1. Mean absolute error (MAE) values in HU and peak-signal-to-noise ratio (PSNR) between synthesized and real CT images when using CycleGAN and UC-GAN model.

	MAE		PSNR	
	CycleGAN	UC-GAN	CycleGAN	UC-GAN
Patient 1	89.7	75.4	45.2	46.1
Patient 2	96.8	81.5	44.1	44.6
Patient 3	94.5	76.7	46.6	47.6
Patient 4	98.9	72.5	45.3	46.1
Patient 5	90.4	78.2	45.0	45.8
Patient 6	93.8	75.6	44.6	46.3
Average ± SD	94.0 ± 4.3	76.7 ± 4.5	45.1 ± 1.5	46.1 ± 1.5

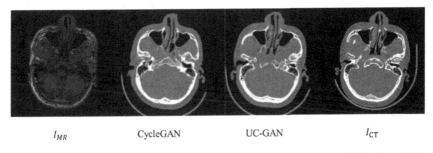

I_{MR} CycleGAN   UC-GAN I_{CT}

Fig. 3. From left to right input MR image, synthesized CT image using CycleGAN, synthesized CT image using UC-GAN, reference real CT image.

A paired t-test on the results in Table 1 shows that for images obtained using the conventional CycleGAN model, the consistency with the reference CT image is significantly lower than that obtained with our proposed UC-GAN model ($p < 0.01$). Figure 3 shows a visual comparison of the results obtained using CycleGAN and UC-GAN. Images obtained using CycleGAN are more blurred and less effective in reconstructing the internal bone structure of the brain.

4   Conclusion and Discussion

In this paper, we combine an improved U-Net network with the CycleGAN model, and improve the image synthesis performance of the CycleGAN architecture, which proves that the performance of CycleGAN model can be further improved.

In our experiments, the parameters were random for each data augmentation, therefore, the data we used for training was actually unpaired. In practical clinical applications, patients typically only accept one scan of a single anatomical region. In this case, there is very little paired data, but there are many different forms of single scan data, which are usually unpaired. Our experimental results show that the proposed model is able to be well applied to the case of unpaired data sets and has practical value.

Although the current synthetic effects have surpassed state-of-the-art method, there is still much room for improvement in the model. For instance, in our model, 2D slices were used for training, and the image's 3D structure information was not used at all, which can be improved in the future work. Also, in practical applications, we tend to pay attention to the specific structure of the image, such as plastic surgeons, will pay more attention to the bone structure of the patient, which requires us to have higher synthetic precision for specific structures. Either we adjust the weight of the corresponding voxel in the image, or we just add the specific structure we want to the model training while setting the other structure of the image as the background.

A combination of U-Net and CycleGAN was proposed to improve the image synthesis performance. Further work will be put on improve critical bone tissue synthesis performance.

Acknowledgments. This work was supported in part by Shenzhen Key Basic Science Program (JCYJ20170413162213765 and JCYJ20180507182437217), the Shenzhen Key Laboratory Program (ZDSYS201707271637577), the NSFC-Shenzhen Union Program (U1613221), and the National Key Research and Development Program (2017YFC0110903).

References

1. Edmund, J.M., Nyholm, T.: A review of substitute CT generation for MRI-only radiation therapy. Radiat. Oncol. **12**(1), 28 (2017)
2. Huo, Y., et al.: SynSeg-Net: synthetic segmentation without target modality ground truth. IEEE Trans. Med. Imag. **38**(4), 1016–1025 (2018)
3. Dowling, J.A., et al.: An atlas-based electron density mapping method for magnetic resonance imaging (MRI)-alone treatment planning and adaptive MRI-based prostate radiation therapy. Int. J. Radiat. Oncol. Biol. Phys. **83**(1), e5–e11 (2012)
4. Chin, A.L., Lin, A., Anamalayil, S., Teo, B.K.: Feasibility and limitations of bulk density assignment in MRI for head and neck IMRT treatment planning. J. Appl. Clin. Med. Phys. **15**(5), 100–111 (2014)
5. Van Nguyen, V., Zhou, K., Vemulapalli, R.: Cross-domain synthesis of medical images using efficient location-sensitive deep network. In: Navab, N., Hornegger, J., Wells, W.M., Frangi, A.F. (eds.) MICCAI 2015, Part I. LNCS, vol. 9349, pp. 677–684. Springer, Heidelberg (2015)
6. Kapanen, M., Tenhunen, M.: T1/T2*-weighted MRI provides clinically relevant pseudo-CT density data for the pelvic bones in MRI-only based radiotherapy treatment planning. Acta Oncol. **52**(3), 612–618 (2013)
7. Johansson, A., Karlsson, M., Nyholm, T.: CT substitute derived from MRI sequences with ultrashort echo time. Med. Phys. **38**(5), 2708–2714 (2011)

8. Zheng, W., Kim, J.P., Kadbi, M., Movsas, B., Chetty, I.J., Glide-Hurst, C.K.: Magnetic resonance-based automatic air segmentation for generation of synthetic computed tomography scans in the head region. Int. J. Radiat. Oncol. Biol. Phys. **93**(3), 497–506 (2015)

9. Sevetlidis, V., Giuffrida, M.V., Tsaftaris, S.A.: Whole image synthesis using a deep encoder-decoder network. In: Tsaftaris, S.A., Gooya, A., Frangi, A.F., Prince, J.L. (eds.) SASHIMI 2016. LNCS, vol. 9968, pp. 127–137. Springer, Cham (2016). https://doi.org/10.1007/978-3-319-46630-9_13

10. Xiang, L., et al.: Deep embedding convolutional neural network for synthesizing CT image from T1-Weighted MR image. Med. Image Anal. **47**, 31–44 (2018)

11. Goodfellow, I., et al.: Generative adversarial nets. In: Advances in Neural Information Processing Systems, pp. 2672–2680 (2014)

12. Nie, D., et al.: Medical image synthesis with context-aware generative adversarial networks. In: Descoteaux, M., Maier-Hein, L., Franz, A., Jannin, P., Collins, D.L., Duchesne, S. (eds.) MICCAI 2017. LNCS, vol. 10435, pp. 417–425. Springer, Cham (2017). https://doi.org/10.1007/978-3-319-66179-7_48

13. Yi, Z., Zhang, H., Tan, P., Gong, M.: DualGAN: unsupervised dual learning for image-to-image translation. In: 2017 IEEE ICCV, pp. 2849–2857. IEEE (2017)

14. Zhu, J.Y., Park, T., Isola, P., Efros, A.A.: Unpaired image-to-image translation using cycle-consistent adversarial networks. In: 2017 IEEE ICCV, pp. 2223–2232. IEEE (2017)

15. Han, X.: MR-based synthetic CT generation using a deep convolutional neural network method. Med. Phys. **44**(4), 1408–1419 (2017)

16. Nie, D., Cao, X., Gao, Y., Wang, L., Shen, D.: Estimating CT image from MRI data using 3D fully convolutional networks. In: Carneiro, G., et al. (eds.) Deep Learning and Data Labeling for Medical Applications, pp. 170–178. Springer, Cham (2016)

17. Wolterink, J.M., Dinkla, A.M., Savenije, M.H., Seevinck, P.R., van den Berg, C.A.T., Išgum, I.: Deep MR to CT synthesis using unpaired data. In: International Workshop on Simulation and Synthesis in Medical Imaging, pp. 14–23 (2017)

18. Ronneberger, O., Fischer, P., Brox, T.: U-Net: convolutional networks for biomedical image segmentation. In: Navab, N., Hornegger, J., Wells, W.M., Frangi, A.F. (eds.) MICCAI 2015. LNCS, vol. 9351, pp. 234–241. Springer, Cham (2015). https://doi.org/10.1007/978-3-319-24574-4_28

19. Jin, C.B., et al.: Deep CT to MR synthesis using paired and unpaired data. Sensors (Basel) **19**(10), E2361 (2019)

20. Kingma, D.P., Ba, J.: Adam: a method for stochastic optimization. In: International Conference on Learning Representations (ICLR) (2015)

CBCT-Based Synthetic MRI Generation for CBCT-Guided Adaptive Radiotherapy

Yang Lei, Tonghe Wang, Joseph Harms, Yabo Fu, Xue Dong,
Walter J. Curran, Tian Liu, and Xiaofeng Yang$^{(\boxtimes)}$

Department of Radiation Oncology and Winship Cancer Institute,
Emory University, Atlanta, GA 30322, USA
xiaofeng.yang@emory.edu

Abstract. Cone-beam computed tomography (CBCT) has been widely used in image-guided radiation therapy for patient setup to improve treatment performance. However, the low soft tissue contrast on CBCT may limit its utility when soft tissue alignment is of interest. Moreover, the potential application of CBCT in adaptive radiation therapy also requires superior soft tissue contrast for online target and organ-at-risk delineation and localization. The purpose of this study is to develop a deep learning-based approach to generate synthetic MRI (sMRI) from CBCT to provide a high soft tissue contrast on CBCT anatomy. The proposed method integrates a dense block and self-attention concept into a cycle-consistent adversarial network (cycleGAN) framework, called attention-cycleGAN, to learn a mapping between CBCT images and paired MRI. Compared with a GAN, a cycleGAN includes an inverse transformation from CBCT to MRI, which constrains the model by forcing a one-to-one mapping. A fully convolution neural network (FCN) with U-Net architecture is used in the generator to enable end-to-end CBCT-to-MRI transformations. Dense blocks and self-attention strategy are used to learn the information to well represent the CBCT image and to map to the specific MRI structure. The experimental results demonstrated that the proposed method could accurately generate sMRI with a similar soft-tissue contract as real MRI.

Keywords: Cone-beam computed tomography · Synthetic MRI · Deep learning

1 Introduction

Cone-beam computed tomography (CBCT) has been widely used in image-guided radiation therapy for prostate cancer patients to improve treatment performance [1, 2]. In current clinical practice, a CBCT is acquired before treatment delivery and provides detailed anatomic information in the treatment position [3, 4]. The displacement of anatomic landmarks between CBCT images and the treatment planning CT images are then measured to quantitatively determine the error in patient setup [5].

In recent years, adaptive radiation therapy has been shown as a promising strategy to improve clinical outcomes by accommodating the inter-fraction variations [6]. In an adaptive radiation therapy workflow, CBCT plays an important role in providing the latest three-dimensional information of patient position and anatomy [7]. More

D. Nguyen et al. (Eds.): AIRT 2019, LNCS 11850, pp. 154–161, 2019.
https://doi.org/10.1007/978-3-030-32486-5_19

demanding applications of CBCT have been proposed, such as daily estimation of target coverage and organs-at-risk (OARs) sparing for real-time CBCT-based treatment replanning [8, 9].

These potential uses of CBCT require accurate and fast delineation of targets and OARs. Experienced physicians are able to manually contour multiple organs on CBCT images, but this is impractical in adaptive radiation therapy due to time constraints. Alternatively, it has been proposed that contours on planning CT images can be propagated to CBCT images by image registration [10]. However, large local variations in patient anatomy and image content between CBCT and CT images is common, e.g. changes in bladder/rectum filling status in prostate cancer patients, and swelling or tumor shrinkage in head-and-neck cancer patients. Such variations are not readily handled by rigid image registration, and not by deformable image registration because of the lack of an exact correspondence of image content between the two image sets. The suboptimal registration result would lead to degraded accuracy of the propagated contours.

Automatic segmentation solely based on CBCT can avoid registration to the planning CT, but very few studies have been published. The contrast of some organs, such as the prostate, is poor on CBCT images. Furthermore, CBCT artifacts caused by scatter contamination degrade image quality [2]. Recently, MRI has been used to aid prostate delineation due to its superior soft tissue contrast, but the corresponding prostate contour needs to be registered to CT images for dose calculation [11–16]. In this study, we propose a novel method to synthesize sMRIs from CBCT images to provide superior soft-tissue contrast. The method includes a deep attention network and several dense blocks to automatically capture the significant features to well represent the CBCT image and to map the MRI. With this sMRI-aided strategy, we can further develop an automated and accurate segmentation method benefiting from the high soft-tissue contrast of MRIs. Our method was evaluated in a retrospective study with 25 head-and-neck patients and 25 pelvic patients.

2   Methods

Section 2.1 begins by describing a system overview of the proposed attention-cycleGAN model and the pre-processing steps to prepare training datasets. In Sect. 2.2, we detail the network architecture of the proposed model. The network losses were described in Sect. 2.3.

2.1   Training and Testing Data and System Overview

The CBCT images of pelvic patients were acquired using the Varian On-Board Imager CBCT system, with voxel size of 0.908 mm $\times$ 0.908 mm $\times$ 2.0 mm. The MR images of pelvic patients were acquired using a Siemens standard MRI scanner with 3D T2-SPACE sequence and $1.0 \times 1.0 \times 2.0$ mm^3 voxel size (TR/TE: 1000/123 ms). The CBCT images of head and neck patients were acquired using the Varian On-Board Imager CBCT system, with imaging spacing of 0.57 mm $\times$ 0.57 mm $\times$ 2.0 mm. The MR images of head and neck patients were acquired using a Siemens MRI scanner with standard T1-weighted SE sequence and $1.2 \times 1.2 \times 2.0$ mm^3 voxel size (TR/TE: 7.3/2.3 ms). Five-fold cross-validation experiment was used to evaluate the proposed method's performance. The training MR and CBCT images were rigidly registered using commercial software, Velocity AI 3.2.1 (Varian Medical Systems, Palo Alto, CA).

Figure 1 illustrates our method's training and synthesis workflow. The proposed algorithm consists of a training stage and a synthesis stage. The deformed MRI was used as the learning-based target of the planning CBCT image for our proposed sMRI-aided strategy. Since the CBCT image is often contaminated with artifacts and small mismatches between MRI even after rigid registration, training a CBCT-to-MRI transformation model is highly under-constrained, meaning small data errors will be amplified during the transformation. In addition, because the two image modalities have fundamentally different properties, training a CBCT-to-MRI transformation model is difficult. To cope with this challenge, 3D cycleGAN architecture was used to learn this transformation model [1, 17]. A cycleGAN framework was used due to its ability to enforce the model to mimic the target data distribution by incorporating an inverse transformation. This helps enforce both anatomical and quantitative accuracy as well as enhancing image contrast. In order to accurately predict each voxel in the anatomic region, we introduced several dense blocks to capture multi-scale information (including low-frequency structural information and high-frequency textural information) by extracting features from previous and following hidden layers. Attention gates (AGs) were used to capture the significant features to well represent the CBCT image.

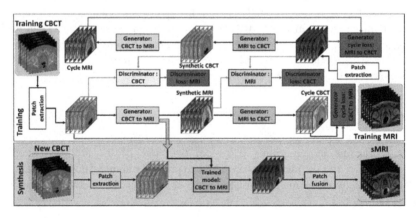

Fig. 1. The schematic flow diagram of the proposed method. The upper row shows the training stage for synthetic MRI inference. The lower row shows the synthesis stage of a new arrival CBCT image.

The proposed attention-cycleGAN model was designed in a 3D patch-based fashion. The training data were collected via extracting pairs of 3D patches by sliding a window with size of $64 \times 64 \times 64$ voxels from paired CBCT and MRI. To enlarge the variety of training data, the overlap between two neighboring patches was set to

$32 \times 32 \times 32$ voxels. This overlap ensures that a continuous whole-image output can be obtained and allows for increased training data for the network.

After training the model, a sMRI of a new patient was obtained by feeding its CBCT patches into the trained model to estimate the sMRI patches, then fusing the sMRI patches together to reconstruct the whole sMRI image. In regions of patch overlap, the final reconstructed voxel value was obtained by averaging the voxel values between the two patches.

2.2 Network Architecture

The proposed network has four separate sub-networks with two generators dedicated for MRI and CBCT synthesis and two discriminators dedicated to measuring whether images it sees are real or synthetic. Figure 2 shows the architectures for these networks.

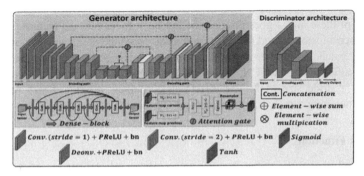

Fig. 2. The architecture of proposed attention cycleGANs including generator and discriminator.

The basic architecture of the generator is a U-Net architecture with several dense blocks and AGs incorporated at the long skip connection. The U-Net architecture consists of an encoding path and a decoding path; the two paths are connected by several long skip connections. In our study, the long skip connection concatenated the feature maps from the current two decoding deconvolution operators and one previous encoding convolution operator by using AGs. Such concatenation with AGs encouraged the network to identify the most relevant semantic contextual information without a requirement to enlarge the receptive field, which might be beneficial for organ localization.

AGs have been explored in the context of semantic segmentation. Previous works demonstrated that the most relevant semantic contextual information can be captured by integrating AGs into a standard U-Net without the need to use a very large reception field. In this study, we incorporated AGs into the design of our generator. Figure 2 shows that AGs were used to implement the skip connection between layers of the encoding path and decoding path. Instead of connecting feature maps with same matrix sizes, as in a standard U-Net, AGs connect feature maps of adjacent layers from different pathways to learn the differences between feature maps. The AGs act immediately prior to the concatenation in order to retain only relevant activations and remove irrelevant/noisy responses. Additionally, AGs filtered the neuron activations during both the forward and backward passes. Gradients originating from image background regions were down weighted during the backward pass. This allows model parameters in shallower layers to be updated based on spatial regions that are most relevant to a given task. AGs also highlighted the most salient features from the encoding path and passed those features through the bridge path.

Several dense blocks were also used for the long skip connection. Dense blocks were used to capture multi-scale information (including low-frequency and high-frequency) by extracting features from the previous and the successive hidden layers and combined these features by short term skip connections between these hidden layers. The dense block is implemented by six convolution layers. A first layer is applied to the input to create k feature maps, which are concatenated to the input. A second layer is then applied to create another k feature maps, which are again concatenated to the previous feature maps. The operation is repeated five times. Then the output of these layers goes through the last layer to shorten the feature maps to k.

The discriminator is used to judge the realism of synthetic image patch against the real image patch. As shown in the discriminator architecture, the discriminator is a typical classification-based FCN, which consists of multiple convolution layers, each of which has a stride size of 2. The discriminator outputs a reduced size patch with element 1 denoting a real voxel and element 0 denoting a fake voxel.

2.3   Loss Functions

As described above, the network relies on continuous improvement of a generator network and a discriminator network. The accuracy of both networks is directly dependent on the design of their corresponding loss functions.

The generator loss function in this study consists of two losses: one is the adversarial loss to distinguish real images from synthetic images; the other is the distance loss to measure the distance between real and synthetic images or between real and cycle images. A weighted summation of the two losses forms the compound loss function for the proposed method:

$$G = \text{argmin}_G\{\lambda_{adv}L_{adv}(G(Y)) + \lambda_{distance}L_{distance}(G(Y), Y)\} \qquad (1)$$

where L_{adv} and $L_{distance}$ are the adversarial loss and the distance loss, λ_{adv} and $\lambda_{distance}$ are balancing parameters of these two losses, Y is the target image and $Z = G(Y)$ is the synthetic image. Distance loss $L_{distance}(Z, Y)$ consists of l_p-norm of the difference image between Z and Y, and the gradient difference (GD) between the two images. The l_p-norm ($p = 1.5$) distance, termed mean p distance (MPD) was introduced to overcome the limitations of the l_1-norm and l_2-norm distance loss such as misclassification by mean absolute distance (MAD) and blurry images by mean squared distance (MSD). Our method can retain image sharpness through minimizing the difference in the magnitude of the gradient between the estimated image and the ground-truth MRI. In this way, the sMRI will try to keep zones with high soft-tissue contrast, such as edges, effectively compensating for the distance loss term.

3   Results

Five-fold cross-validation testing was performed on 25 head and neck and 25 pelvic patients' CBCT/MRI datasets. We randomly partitioned the 25 patient images into five equal sized subgroups. One subgroup was retained as the validation data for testing the model, and the remaining four subgroups were used as the training data. Normalized mean absolute error (NMAE), peak signal-to-noise ratio (PSNR) and normalized cross correlation (NCC) were calculated between the deformed and fixed images for quantitative evaluations.

Figure 3 shows axial views of the pelvic CBCT image, MRI and sMRIs, and deformed prostate manual contours at two axial levels for a patient. To better illustrate the contrast enhancement of sMRI-aided strategy, Fig. 3 (a5) compare the profiles of the dashed blue line in subfigures (a4) for CT image, MRI and sMRIs. The dashed line passing through the bladder, prostate, and rectum manual contours was set to 0 if the voxel was outside of one of the contours, and 1.1 for the voxels within the organs. Thus, the boundary of the prostate is the discontinuity on the plot profile. To provide a meaningful comparison, we use a $\frac{x-\min(X)}{\max(X)-\min(X)}$ normalization to scale voxel intensities on the dash line to $[0, 1]$, where x denotes a voxel's intensity on dash line, X denotes the all voxels' intensity appeared on dashed line. As is shown in subfigure (a5), sMRI provides superior bladder and prostate contrast to CBCT image, similar to that of conventional MR image. Figure 4 shows the axial views of sMRI result for a head and neck patient. As can be seen from Fig. 4, the contrast around spinal cord region was enhanced. Overall, the mean NMAE, PSNR and NCC were 0.06 ± 0.03, 19.8 ± 2.6 dB and 0.85 ± 0.09 for pelvic site, and were 0.05 ± 0.02, 20.2 ± 3.7 dB and 0.87 ± 0.07 for head and neck site (Table 1).

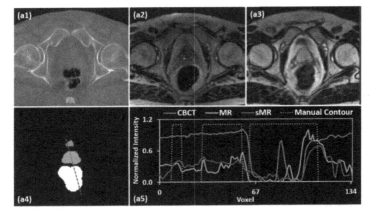

Fig. 3. Visual results of generated sMRI. (a1) shows the original CBCT image at axial level, (a2) shows the corresponding MR image, (a3) shows the generated sMRI, (a4) shows the deformed manual contour, (a5) shows the plot profile of CT, MRI, sMRI, and manual contour of the blue dashed line in (a1), respectively. (Color figure online)

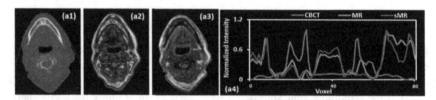

Fig. 4. Visual results of generated sMRI. (a1) shows the original CBCT image at axial level, (a2) shows the corresponding MR image, (a3) shows the generated sMRI, (a4) shows the plot profile of CT, MRI and sMRI of the blue dashed line in (a2), respectively. (Color figure online)

Table 1. Numerical evaluation of the proposed method.

	Pelvic			Head & Neck		
	NMAE	PSNR (dB)	NCC	NMAE	PSNR (dB)	NCC
Proposed	0.06 ± 0.03	19.8 ± 2.6	0.85 ± 0.09	0.05 ± 0.02	20.2 ± 3.7	0.87 ± 0.07

4   Conclusion and Discussion

The method proposed can be used for generating sMRI from daily CBCT. This study demonstrated that the proposed methods are capable of reliably generating sMRI with high soft-tissue contrast, which could be helpful for accurate target and OAR delineation and localization for adaptive dose planning, then warrant further development of a CBCT-guided adaptive radiotherapy workflow. The utilization of sMRI can also be used for CBCT/MRI cross modality registration.

Acknowledgements. This research is supported in part by the National Cancer Institute of the National Institutes of Health under Award Number R01CA215718, and Dunwoody Golf Club Prostate Cancer Research Award, a philanthropic award provided by the Winship Cancer Institute of Emory University.

Disclosure: The authors declare no conflicts of interest.

References

1. Harms, J., et al.: Paired cycle-GAN-based image correction for quantitative cone-beam computed tomography. Med. Phys. **46**, 3998–4009 (2019)
2. Lei, Y., et al.: Learning-based CBCT correction using alternating random forest based on auto-context model. Med. Phys. **46**(2), 601–618 (2019)
3. Hvid, C.A., Elstrom, U.V., Jensen, K., Grau, C.: Cone-beam computed tomography (CBCT) for adaptive image guided head and neck radiation therapy. Acta Oncol. **57**(4), 552–556 (2018)
4. Yang, X., et al.: A learning-based method to improve pelvis cone beam CT image quality for prostate cancer radiation therapy. Int. J. Radiat. Oncol. Biol. Phys. **102**(3), e377–e378 (2018)

5. Barney, B.M., Lee, R.J., Handrahan, D., Welsh, K.T., Cook, J.T., Sause, W.T.: Image-guided radiotherapy (IGRT) for prostate cancer comparing kV imaging of fiducial markers with cone beam computed tomography (CBCT). Int. J. Radiat. Oncol. Biol. Phys. **80**(1), 301–305 (2011)

6. Kataria, T., et al.: Clinical outcomes of adaptive radiotherapy in head and neck cancers. Br. J. Radiol. **89**(1062), 20160085 (2016)

7. Oldham, M., et al.: Cone-beam-CT guided radiation therapy: a model for on-line application. Radiother. Oncol. J. Eur. Soc. Ther. Radiol. Oncol. **75**(3), 271–278 (2005)

8. Yoo, S., Yin, F.: Dosimetric feasibility of cone-beam CT-based treatment planning compared to CT-based treatment planning. Int. J. Radiat. Oncol. Biol. Phys. **66**(5), 1553–1561 (2006)

9. de la Zerda, A., Armbruster, B., Xing, L.: Formulating adaptive radiation therapy (ART) treatment planning into a closed-loop control framework. Phys. Med. Biol. **52**(14), 4137–4153 (2007)

10. Thor, M., Petersen, J.B., Bentzen, L., Hoyer, M., Muren, L.P.: Deformable image registration for contour propagation from CT to cone-beam CT scans in radiotherapy of prostate cancer. Acta Oncol. **50**(6), 918–925 (2011)

11. Yang, X., et al.: Pseudo CT estimation from MRI using patch-based random forest. In: Proceedings of SPIE, pp. 101332Q (2017)

12. Yang, X., et al.: A learning-based approach to derive electron density from anatomical MRI for radiation therapy treatment planning. Int. J. Radiat. Oncol. **99**(2), S173–S174 (2017)

13. Wang, T., et al.: MRI-based treatment planning for brain stereotactic radiosurgery: dosimetric validation of a learning-based pseudo-CT generation method. Med. Dosim. Official J. Am. Assoc. Med. Dosimetrists **44**, 199–204 (2019)

14. Lei, Y., et al.: MRI-based pseudo CT synthesis using anatomical signature and alternating random forest with iterative refinement model. J. Med. Imaging. **5**(4), 043504 (2018)

15. Yang, X., et al.: MRI-Based synthetic CT for radiation treatment of prostate cancer. Int. J. Radiat. Oncol. **102**(3), S193–S194 (2018)

16. Shafai-Erfani, G., et al.: Dose evaluation of MRI-based synthetic CT generated using a machine learning method for prostate cancer radiotherapy. Med. Dosim. Official J. Am. Assoc. Med. Dosimetrists (2019, in press)

17. Lei, Y., et al.: MRI-only based synthetic CT generation using dense cycle consistent generative adversarial networks. Med. Phys. **46**(8), 3565–3581 (2019)

Cardio-Pulmonary Substructure Segmentation of CT Images Using Convolutional Neural Networks

Rabia Haq[1]([✉]), Alexandra Hotca[2], Aditya Apte[1], Andreas Rimner[2], Joseph O. Deasy[1], and Maria Thor[1]

[1] Department of Medical Physics, Memorial Sloan-Kettering Cancer Center, New York, NY 10017, USA
{haqr,aptea,deasyj,thorm}@mskcc.org
[2] Department of Radiation Oncology, Memorial Sloan-Kettering Cancer Center, New York, NY 10017, USA
{hotcacha,rimnera}@mskcc.org

Abstract. Radiotherapy doses to some cardio-pulmonary substructures may be critical factors in the observed early mortality following radiotherapy for nonsmall cell lung cancer patients. Our goal is to provide an open-source tool to automatically segment cardio-vascular substructures for consistent outcomes analyses, and subsequently for radiation treatment planning of thoracic patients. Here, we built and validated a multi-label Deep Learning Segmentation (DLS) framework for accurate auto-segmentation of cardio-pulmonary substructures. The DLS framework utilized a deep neural network architecture to segment 12 cardio-pulmonary substructures from Computed Tomography (CT) scans of 217 patients previously treated with thoracic RT. The model was robust against variability in image quality characteristics, including the presence/absence of contrast. A hold-out dataset of additional 24 CT scans was used for quantitative evaluation of the final model against expert contours using Dice Similarity Coefficients (DSC) and 95th Percentile of Hausdorff Distance (HD95). DLS contours of an additional 10 CT scans were reviewed by a radiation oncologist to determine the number of slices in need of adjustment for each of the non-overlapping substructures. The DLS model reduced segmentation time per patient from about one hour of manual segmentation to 10 s. Quantitatively, the highest accuracy was observed for the Heart (median DSC $= (0.96(0.91 - 0.93))$ and HD95 $= (4.3\,\mathrm{mm}(3.8\,\mathrm{mm} - 5.5\,\mathrm{mm}))$. The median DSC for the remaining structures was $0.80 - 0.92$. The expert judged that, on average, 85% of the contours were equivalent to state-of-the-art manual contouring and did not require any modifications.

Keywords: Semantic segmentation · Convolutional neural networks · Cardio-pulmonary · Radiation therapy

© Springer Nature Switzerland AG 2019
D. Nguyen et al. (Eds.): AIRT 2019, LNCS 11850, pp. 162–169, 2019.
https://doi.org/10.1007/978-3-030-32486-5_20

1   Introduction

Various studies have shown that doses to some cardio-vascular substructures may be critical factors in the observed heart toxicity and early mortality following radiotherapy (RT) for nonsmall cell lung cancer (NSCLC) [10,14–16]. This may be attributed to irradiation of particular constituents of the cardio-pulmonary system. Currently, segmentation of cardio-pulmonary organs other than the whole heart and lung has been overlooked, and only these two organs are routinely defined as part of the treatment planning process. RT planning requires robust and accurate segmentation of organs-at-risk in order to maximize radiation to the disease location and to spare the normal tissue as much as possible. The introduction of a new set of organs puts requirements on both segmentation accuracy and segmentation time that would result in an overhead of several hours of manual segmentation and contour refinement in the clinic.

We built and validated a multi-label Deep Learning Segmentation (DLS) framework for accurate auto-segmentation of cardio-pulmonary substructures. The DLS framework utilized a deep convolutional neural network architecture to segment 12 cardio-pulmonary substructures [4] from Computed Tomography (CT) scans of 217 patients previously treated with thoracic RT. The segmented substructures are: Heart, Pericardium, Atria, Ventricles, Aorta, Left Atrium (LA), Right Atrium (RA), Left Ventricle (LA), Right Ventricle (RV), Inferior Vena Cava (IVC), Superior Vena Cava (SVC) and Pulmonary Artery (PA). We evaluate our framework using a hold-out dataset of 24 CT scans by calculating quantitative as well as qualitative validation metrics. A radiation oncologist qualitatively evaluated auto-generated contours for an additional set of 10 CT scans to determine that, on average, 85% of the non-overlapping substructure contours required no modifications and were acceptable for clinical use.

2   Methodology

Our approach utilizes deep neural network for 2D segmentation of contrast as well as non-contrast enhanced thoracic CT images. The network auto-crops input CT scans around the lungs to extract the region of interest. The network is trained to perform multi-label prediction of eight non-overlapping, contiguous substructures, which are: aorta, LA, LV, RA, RV, IVC, SVC and PA. Additionally it is individually trained to segment the overlapping structures such as the heart, the atria, pericardium and ventricles. Output label predictions for the multi-label segmentation network and overlapping structures were combined for each input scan, resulting in auto-segmentation of 12 cardio-pulmonary substructures.

2.1   Experimental Datasets

Experimental data consisted of CT scans of 241 patients obtained from our institutional clinic. This data consisted of contrast as well as non-contrast enhanced images of varying imaging quality and resolution across different scanners. Manual expert segmentation for 12 organs-at-risk cardio-pulmonary structures was considered ground truth and used for model training, testing and validation. 192 CT scans were utilized for model training, 24 CT scans were used for model testing and the remaining 24 CT scans were used for hold-out validation respectively. These scans were auto-cropped around the lungs to extract the volume of interest around the heart substructures. 2D axial slices pertaining to each patient image volume were resized to 512×512 and normalized, resulting in a total of 10,284 training images. Network input data was augmented per batch and consisted of random cropping, random horizontal and vertical flipping and rotation by ten degrees. Resulting auto-segmented 2D axial images were stacked back together to generate 3D segmentations without further post-processing.

An additional dataset of 10 RT planning thoracic CT scans, for which no expert contours were available, was used for qualitative contour evaluation by a radiologist to determine auto-generated contour acceptability for clinical use.

2.2   Network Architecture

Our approach, as depicted in Fig. 1 leveraged the deep neural network architecture of [1]. Convolutional neural networks (CNNs) and encoder-decoder neural networks have been successfully employed for medical image segmentation tasks [6, 7, 12, 13]. The Deeplab encoder-decoder network architecture with atrous separable convolutions consists of spatial pyramid pooling that encodes multi-scale contextual information to capture spatial anatomical information of contiguous structures. Dense feature maps extracted in the last encoder network path consist of detailed semantic information. The decoder network was able to robustly recover structure boundaries through bilinear upsampling at a factor of 4 while applying atrous convolutions to reduce features before semantic labeling. We trained the network using ResNet-101 [5] as the encoder network backbone with learning rate $= 0.01$ using "policy" learning rate scheduler [8], crop size $= 513 \times 513$, batch size $= 8$, loss $=$ cross-entropy, output stride $= 16$ for 50 epochs for dense label prediction. Our approach has been implemented using the Pytorch DL framework.

We also investigated the performance of various network loss functions and their influence on correct multi-label prediction. We trained our network with various segmentation losses on the same architecture backbone to account for varying structure sizes and class imbalance during training and determine the efficacy of modifying label prediction probabilities during back propagation for multi-label segmentation. The network was trained using cross entropy (CE), Multi-class Dice Loss (M-DSC), Generalized Dice Loss (G-DSC) [11] and a weighted combination of (0.5G-DSC + 0.5CE) which pixel-wise CE resulting in superior segmentation performance. Cross entropy loss can be described as

$$L(\chi; \theta) = -\sum_{x \in \chi} \log p(t_i | x_i; \theta), \tag{1}$$

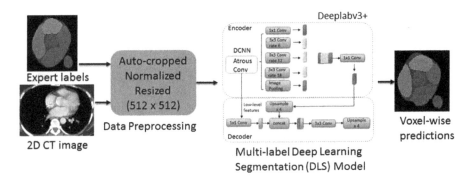

Fig. 1. Schematic overview of the proposed deep learning multi-label segmentation scheme. The network is trained on 2D CT images that are auto-cropped around the lung region of interest, augmented and batch normalized for dense label prediction.

where X denotes the input images, $p(t_i|x_i; \theta)$ is the pixel probability of the target class $x_i \in \chi$ that is being predicted with network parameters θ. A quantitative comparison of auto-segmentation results using the aforementioned various network losses can be found in Table 3.

2.3   Model Evaluation

We quantitatively evaluated the auto-generated segmentations by comparing the Dice Coefficient (DSC) and 95th Percentile Hausdorff Distance (HD95 (mm)) of 24 patients against expert clinical segmentations. Additionally, an expert qualitatively evaluated the auto-generated multi-label segmentations for an additional cohort of 10 thoracic CT scans to validate the clinical usability of the auto-contours. No expert contours were present for this additional validation dataset. The expert reviewed substructure contours on axial slices of the CT images and rated them on a four-grade score: Good (requiring no adjustments), Acceptable (acceptable auto-contour deviations), Need of Adjustments (NOA) and Poor (requiring larger number of slice adjustments). Rating was performed by listing the number of slices requiring contour adjustments in relation to the

Table 1. Criteria for scoring each cardiac substructure contour in clinical scoring, showing the number of CT image slices, and percentage of extended structures, that need to be unapproved due to minor modifications for each grade. NOA: Need of Adjustments.

Scoring	IVC	SVC, PA, LA, LV, RA, RV	Aorta
Good	0 slices (0%)	0 slices (0%)	0 slices (0%)
Acceptable	1–3 slices (up to 18%)	1–5 slices (up to 17%)	1–10 slices (up to 16%)
NOA	4–5 slices (up to 29%)	6–8 slices (up to 27%)	11–14 slices (up to 22%)
Poor	>5 slices (>29%)	>8 slices (>27%)	>14 slices (>22%)

average number of slices spanning each substructure. Criteria for the clinical contour scoring is presented in Table 1.

3   Results and Discussion

Table 2 compares the DSC evaluation metric for segmentations using the network training loss cross-entropy (CE) against other network training losses. Our experiments demonstrated that pixel-wise target class loss calculation using CE resulted in improved multi-label segmentation predictions when compared against Multi-class Dice Loss (M-DSC), Generalized Dice Loss (G-DSC) and a weighted combination of (0.5CE + 0.5G-DSC). Although the DSC score for Aorta, which is the largest substructure during multi-label segmentation, is improved as expected using the G-DSC loss, the accuracy of smaller, tubular substructures was reduced.

Table 2. Multi-label segmentation comparison of eight cardio-pulmonary substructures between various network training loss configurations using the DSC evaluation metric. All training losses were implemented using the same network architecture and hyperparameters. Highest achieved accuracies are highlighted in bold.

Network training loss	Aorta	LA	LV	RA	RV	IVC	SVC	PA
Gen. Dice Loss (G-DSC)	**0.90**	**0.86**	**0.92**	**0.85**	0.81	0.61	0.82	0.87
Multi-class Dice Loss (M-DSC)	0.82	**0.86**	**0.92**	0.84	0.86	0.76	0.79	0.86
Combined Loss (G-DSC + CE)	0.81	0.83	0.91	0.81	0.85	0.76	0.80	0.86
Cross Entropy (CE)	0.83	**0.86**	**0.92**	**0.85**	**0.86**	**0.81**	**0.84**	**0.88**

Figure 2 displays the DSC Score results for the 24 hold-out validation CT images for all 12 substructures segmented using the CE loss. Our achieved DSC accuracies are comparable to the state-of-the-art multi-atlas [9] and deep learning methods [3] for segmenting cardio-pulmonary substructures from CT images. The highest segmentation accuracy was observed for the heart (median DSC = 0.96, median HD95 = 3.48 mm), while the remaining structures achieving median accuracy ($0.81 \leq$ DSC ≤ 0.94) and (6 mm $\leq$ HD95 ≤ 3 mm), with highest HD95 surface distance accuracy observed for Aorta. Figure 3 display the qualitative contour results comparing the DLS contours against expert contours.

Table 3 displays the clinical contour evaluation scores of the auto-generated contours for 10 thoracic RT CT scans using the grading criteria described in Table 1. The expert identified all need for adjustments as minor modifications, with contours in acceptable ranges for the IVC, SVC, PA, LA and LV (median adjustments ranging between 5 to 15%). Most required adjustments were observed in the RV, with median 24% contours requiring modifications. Most of the minor adjustments were observed near the superior portion of the

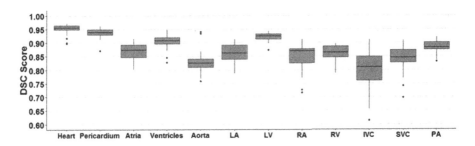

Fig. 2. Dice Similarity Coefficient (DSC) Score results of the 24 thoracic RT CT images comparing the auto-generated DLS contours against the manually segmented expert contours for 12 cardio-pulmonary substructures.

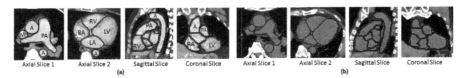

Fig. 3. Comparison of the auto-generated DLS contours (depicted in blue) against the expert delineations (depicted in green) for two patients (a) and (b) in axial, sagittal and coronal plane views. The Aorta, PA and SVC are visible in Axial Slice 1, whereas the four chambers: LA, LV, RA and RV, and the Aorta are visible in Axial Slice 2. A: aorta. (Color figure online)

Table 3. Qualitative evaluation of auto-generated segmentations of 10 thoracic RT patient CT scans. A radiation oncologist expert determined the percentage of each auto-generated structure segmentation in Need of Adjustments (NOA). Expert identified all required changes as minor modifications. Least and most adjustments were required for SVC and RV structures, respectively, for clinical acceptance and use.

% NOA	Aorta	IVC	SVC	PA	LA	LV	RA	RV
Min	13	0	0	0	0	3	8	7
Max	27	59	13	45	34	29	43	47
Median	**19**	**15**	**5**	**12**	**15**	**8**	**20**	**24**

structures between CT image contour transitions. This may be attributed to the image artifacts introduced due to heart motion and image acquisition.

The qualitative scoring and quantitative evaluation for the aorta and IVC is lower than expected because both these substructure segmentations were extended on image slices beyond the clinical contouring protocol. According to the clinical contour guidelines, these two substructures should not be contoured beyond two slices below the last contoured image slice of the heart in the axial plane. However, due to lack of training on a large set of background CT images in the posterior portion of the heart contour during network training, our model continued to segment the aorta and IVC because of the presence of the substructure edges beyond the heart contour. This highlighted the consideration towards additional spatial input data requirements during network training for generating clinically acceptable auto-segmentations as input to radiation treatment planning.

4 Conclusion

We propose a model for auto-segmentation of cardio-pulmonary substructures from contrast and non-contrast enhanced CT images. The proposed model reduced substructure segmentation time for a new patient from about one hour of manual segmentation to approximately 10 s. We demonstrated that the model is robust against variability in image quality characteristics, including the presence or absence of contrast. We validated our approach by quantitatively comparing resulting contours against expert delineation. An expert concluded that overall 85% of the auto-generated contours are acceptable for clinical use without requiring adjustments. The resulting segmentations can effectively be utilized to study the effect of heart toxicity and clinical outcomes, as well as used as input to radiation therapy treatment planning. We have applied our approach to auto-segment an additional 283 treatment planning CT scans to study heart toxicity outcomes for lung cancer. The developed cardio-pulmonary segmentation models have being integrated into deep learning tools within the open-source CERR [2] platform.

Acknowledgments. This research is partially supported by NCI R01 CA198121.

References

1. Chen, L.-C., Zhu, Y., Papandreou, G., Schroff, F., Adam, H.: Encoder-decoder with atrous separable convolution for semantic image segmentation. In: Ferrari, V., Hebert, M., Sminchisescu, C., Weiss, Y. (eds.) ECCV 2018. LNCS, vol. 11211, pp. 833–851. Springer, Cham (2018). https://doi.org/10.1007/978-3-030-01234-2_49
2. Deasy, J., Blanco, A., Clark, V.: CERR: a computational environment for radiotherapy research. Med. Phys. **30**(5), 979–85 (2003)
3. Dormer, J.D., et al.: Heart chamber segmentation from CT using convolutional neural networks. In: Proceedings of SPIE - The International Society for Optical Engineering (2018)
4. Feng, M., Moran, J., Koelling, T., et al.: Development and validation of a heart atlas to study cardiac exposure to radiation following treatment for breast cancer. Int. J. Radiat. Oncol. Biol. Phys. **79**(1), 10–18 (2010)
5. He, K., Zhang, X., Ren, S., Sun, J.: Deep residual learning for image recognition. In: 2016 IEEE Conference on Computer Vision and Pattern Recognition (CVPR), pp. 770–778, June 2016. https://doi.org/10.1109/CVPR.2016.90
6. Isensee, F., et al.: nnU-Net: self-adapting framework for U-Net-based medical image segmentation. CoRR abs/1809.10486 (2018). http://arxiv.org/abs/1809.10486

7. Jin, Q., Meng, Z., Sun, C., Wei, L., Su, R.: RA-UNet: a hybrid deep attention-aware network to extract liver and tumor in CT scans. CoRR abs/1811.01328 (2018). http://arxiv.org/abs/1811.01328

8. Liu, W., Rabinovich, A., Berg, A.C.: ParseNet: looking wider to see better. CoRR abs/1506.04579 (2015). http://arxiv.org/abs/1506.04579

9. Luo, Y., et al.: Automatic segmentation of cardiac substructures from noncontrast CT images: accurate enough for dosimetric analysis? Acta Oncol. **58**(1), 81–87 (2019)

10. McWilliam, A., Kennedy, J., et al.: Radiation dose to heart base linked with poorer survival in lung cancer patients. Eur. J. Cancer **85**, 106–113 (2017)

11. Milletari, F., Navab, N., Ahmadi, S.: V-Net: fully convolutional neural networks for volumetric medical image segmentation. CoRR abs/1606.04797 (2016). http://arxiv.org/abs/1606.04797

12. Oktay, O., et al.: Anatomically constrained neural networks (ACNNs): application to cardiac image enhancement and segmentation. IEEE Trans. Med. Imaging **37**(2), 384–395 (2018)

13. Oktay, O., et al.: Attention U-Net: learning where to look for the pancreas. CoRR abs/1804.03999 (2018). http://arxiv.org/abs/1804.03999

14. Dess, R.T., Sun, Y., et al.: Cardiac events after radiation therapy: combined analysis of prospective multicenter trials for locally advanced non-small-cell lung cancer. J. Clin. Oncol. **35**, 1395–402 (2017)

15. Thor, M., Deasy, J., et al.: The role of heart-related dose-volume metrics on overall survival in the RTOG 0617 clinical trial. Int. J. Radiat. Oncol. Biol. Phys. **102**, S96 (2018)

16. Vivekanandan, S., Landau, D., Counsell, N., Warren, D., Khwanda, A., et al.: The impact of cardiac radiation dosimetry on survival after radiation therapy for non-small cell lung cancer. Int. J. Radiat. Oncol. **99**, 51–60 (2017)

Author Index

Printed in the United States
By Bookmasters